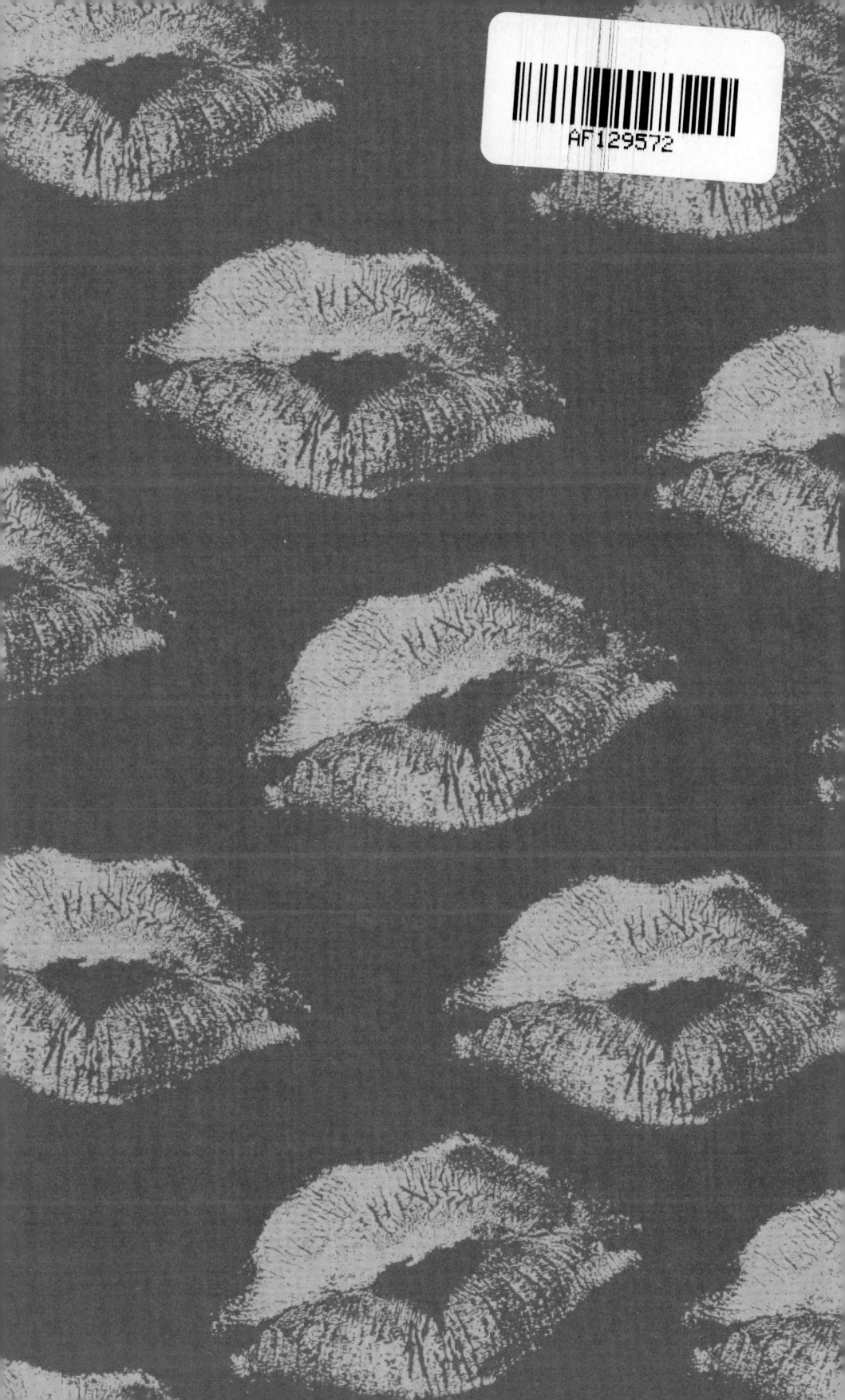

BIMBO

BIMBO

Ditch the Labels. Find Your Voice.
Reclaim Your Confidence.

ASHLEY JAMES

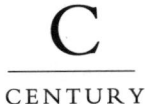

CENTURY

UK | USA | Canada | Ireland | Australia
India | New Zealand | South Africa

Century is part of the Penguin Random House group of companies
whose addresses can be found at global.penguinrandomhouse.com

Penguin Random House UK,
One Embassy Gardens, 8 Viaduct Gardens, London SW11 7BW

penguin.co.uk
global.penguinrandomhouse.com

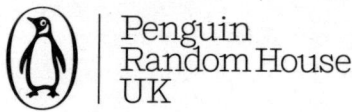

First published 2026
004

Copyright © Ashley James, 2026

The moral right of the author has been asserted

Penguin Random House values and supports copyright. Copyright fuels creativity, encourages diverse voices, promotes freedom of expression and supports a vibrant culture. Thank you for purchasing an authorised edition of this book and for respecting intellectual property laws by not reproducing, scanning or distributing any part of it by any means without permission. You are supporting authors and enabling Penguin Random House to continue to publish books for everyone. No part of this book may be used or reproduced in any manner for the purpose of training artificial intelligence technologies or systems. In accordance with Article 4(3) of the DSM Directive 2019/790, Penguin Random House expressly reserves this work from the text and data mining exception.

Set in 13.4/16pt Bembo Book MT Pro
Typeset by Six Red Marbles UK, Thetford, Norfolk

Printed and bound in Great Britain by Clays Ltd, Elcograf S.p.A.

The authorised representative in the EEA is Penguin Random House Ireland,
Morrison Chambers, 32 Nassau Street, Dublin D02 YH68

A CIP catalogue record for this book is available from the British Library

ISBN: 978-1-529-95877-5

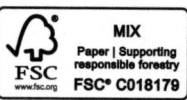

Penguin Random House is committed to a sustainable future for our business, our readers and our planet. This book is made from Forest Stewardship Council® certified paper.

For women.

For the ones who came before us – who fought, sacrificed and endured so that we might have the freedoms we hold today. For those who suffered under oppression, silenced and unseen.

For trans women, our sisters in arms – because none of us are free until we all are. For every woman still fighting for equality.

For all our male allies. We need you as much today as we did yesterday. Thank you for lending your voices to us.

And for our daughters, especially my own – my Ada. May you grow up in a world of equal opportunity, unshackled by double standards, and free to live boldly as yourselves.

CONTENTS

Introduction   1

GIRLHOOD

1. Princess   15
2. Like a Girl   18
3. Bossy Boots   24
4. Fitting In   27
5. 'Tarty-Warty Ashley'   37
6. Aunt Flo   40

MAIDENHOOD

7. 'Not Like the Other Girls'   47
8. Pretty Privilege   52
9. School Slut   59
10. Deflowered   65
11. Mind the Gap (in our Sex Education)   69
12. Schooling in Sexism   71
13. Vulvas for the Win   75
14. Too Much   78
15. Silly Girl   82
16. Beauty or Brains   88

WOMANHOOD

17. Working Girl — 97
18. 'Crazy Ex-Girlfriend' — 101
19. 'She Looks like a Girl from Abercrombie & Fitch' — 105
20. Posh Totty — 108
21. 'I Kissed a Girl (and I Liked It)' — 112
22. Fame Hungry — 117
23. Sex Sells — 120
24. 'Who've You Got the Girls out for?' — 123
25. A Moment on the Lips, a Lifetime on Your Sense of Self-Worth — 130

SINGLEHOOD

26. Running Out of Time — 143
27. Left on the Shelf — 150
28. The Difference Between Lonely and Alone — 159
29. Tick Tock, it's the Biological Clock — 165
30. Decentring Men — 168
31. Silent Sisterhood Shifts — 174
32. Backing the Wrong Pony — 177
33. Learning to Love — 182
34. Girlfriend Material — 188
35. Happily Never After — 195
36. Bride and Prejudice? — 203

MOTHERHOOD

37.	The Mother of All Labels	211
38.	One of 'Those' Mums	217
39.	The Negative Nancys and the Just-You-Waits	221
40.	Mum Wars	224
41.	I'm a Mum's Mum	231
42.	Ruining Your Body	236
43.	Negative Birth Stories	241
44.	The Gender Pain Gap	248
45.	A 'Positive Birth Story'	253
46.	Baby Weight and Bouncing Back	258
47.	Lie Back and Think of England	270
48.	Daddy Day Care and the Mother of All Mental Loads	277
49.	The Bake Sale with a Side of Mum Guilt	288
50.	Crash Landing from Cloud Nine	292
51.	Is it Normal to Regret Motherhood?	297
52.	The Weight of it All	301
53.	Finding Your Pink	304
54.	The Power of Mum	309
55.	Being a Boy Mum	313

ELDERHOOD 319

Conclusion	330
Acknowledgements	337
Notes	339
Reading List	343
Index	345

'Until the lion learns how to write, the story will always glorify the hunter.'

—African proverb

BOSSY / DRAMA QUEEN / ATTENTION SEEKER / DIVA / COW / PRUDE / FRUMPY / FRIGID / COCK-TEASE / TART / SLUT / WHORE / HO / DYKE / PICK-ME GIRL / BIMBO / AIRHEAD / BIRD / POSH TOTTY / CAT LADY / CRAZY / SPINSTER / FEMINAZI / BITCH / GOLD DIGGER / NEEDY / HYSTERICAL / BRIDEZILLA / TROPHY WIFE / WAG / NAG / BALLBUSTER / BALL AND CHAIN / MUMSY / MILF / HOMEWRECKER / COUGAR / BATTLE AXE / MUTTON / WITCH / HAG / MATRON / BIDDY / BINT / CRONE

INTRODUCTION

These are just some of the words we use to keep women and girls in their place. I'm sure I'm not the only one who has been called several of them. And I'm sure I'll hear plenty more as I continue my journey through womanhood into middle and old age, before I'm expected to become invisible.

My daughter Ada is two years old. When I look at her, I see a girl who is confident, loud and proud. A girl who looks at herself in the mirror with love, amazement and wonder. She loves her body. She's not scared to speak her mind and tell us NO. She's happy. When I look at her, I see myself as a child. Because that was me too once. Probably you too. No little girl is born a 'bimbo'. Nor does she arrive into the world as a 'prude', 'bitch' or 'slag'.

So why is it that, by the time we enter our twenties, many of us feel so small? When we look at our bodies, we no longer feel wonder and awe, but shame and worry? We stop feeling comfortable saying no because we worry that will make us unlikeable. We start believing we're not enough on our own and we need to find our 'other half' to be complete. We're taught to downsize ourselves – to be slight, quiet and palatable. I felt like this for most of my teens and adult life, but when I reached twenty-seven, something snapped and I just couldn't take hating myself anymore.

I set off on a journey of self-love and discovery, and started exploring my own path, one that led me to question the outdated labels, rules and expectations placed on women. As I dug deeper into where these pressures come from, I started to uncover more about our history as women and the oppression and injustices our ancestors suffered. So much of our present is also the past, filtered through the expectations placed upon us today. I realised that my insecurities, lack of self-esteem and faltering confidence were so completely wrapped up in the various messages I'd learned about what it means to be a *good* or *attractive* or *acceptable* woman. And perhaps, even more, it was all tangled up with the double standards everywhere in society – with one benchmark for women and an entirely different one for men.

To rediscover my confidence, I had to untie all the knots about womanhood that were eating me up inside. To unlearn anything we've been bred to believe, we first need to understand it. This book will tell the story of how I got there. Spoiler alert: for me, the secret to self-acceptance was feminism.

Have you ever read something on social media, or sat in a group of women or men talking about feminism, and found yourself feeling completely lost? If so, you're not alone. I definitely didn't fully understand it myself for a long time. And much to my embarrassment now, I even held a slightly negative view of feminists and the movement as a whole. Aside from the fact that many feminist messages are drowned out by those in positions of power, over the past 150 years, their message has been twisted and turned upside down successfully by those who want to maintain the status quo. The bra-burning, man-hating feminist caricature is useful because it turns women against their own interests. It makes us feel that feminism is not for us. I certainly didn't identify with the 'feminazis'.

What I've learned, over the years, on my journey from girlhood to womanhood, is that society tries to keep us in all kinds of boxes. And one of the most powerful tools it uses to keep us there is language. Words have the power to shrink us, to shame us, to keep us small. But it's only by breaking free from these pigeonholes and labels, by ditching the stereotypes and expectations, that we can begin to live unapologetically.

Growing up, we were probably all scared of the words in the list at the beginning of this book. But I hope, through reading these pages, you will soon realise that you're *not* a failure if you have been called them. These words are used to police us and to keep us on track re what society calls 'normal' femininity. But not all of us are built to stay on the rails.

I want to challenge some of the norms and traditions, the expectations and milestones, and encourage women to question them too. To push us all to see that we deserve more. I'm sharing my own experiences in the hope that you don't make the same mistakes I have. Or that, if you have, you can feel less alone and stop beating yourself up over them. Whether you're going through a break-up, feeling like the eternally single one, choosing to be child-free, or struggling with the invisibility of motherhood – there's something in these pages for *you*.

Women often message me asking for help finding the words they need to stand up for themselves – whether it's pushing back against the opinions of partners, parents or employers. Often these men and women – the ones being pushed back against – aren't bad people, they just hold on to outdated views about how women should behave. So many of us lack the vocabulary to advocate for ourselves. We certainly weren't taught it in school. Many of us weren't taught it at home either. By telling my stories, I want to help you reclaim your own voice, and hopefully, in doing so, you'll begin to regain the confidence of that little girl you once were – piece by piece.

This book will confront the insults, labels and expectations that women face every day, and show how understanding them and stepping outside of them can lead to a bigger, freer life. While my path is my own, and I fully recognise my privileges, I hope you'll see parallels with your own experiences. I hope you'll begin to spot all the ways the world tries to keep women small, compliant, and afraid to take up space. My main takeaway is that the seemingly endless list of derogatory terms are just easy ways to punch down. You can't win – you're either a 'slut' or a 'prude'. These gendered words are there to keep us in those boxes and make us behave in a way that men find palatable.

Women are *still* constantly pitted against each other. So many of us have internalised the belief that, in order to succeed, we have to one-up each other. It's the same tired binaries: madonna versus whore, mothers versus child-free women, tomboy versus girly girl, too fat or too thin, grow old gracefully or fight the ageing process, Hailey versus Selena . . . Even though we are in a much stronger position socially, culturally and financially than we were a hundred, fifty, even ten years ago, it feels like women's rights are being rolled back around the world. I hope this book is a rallying cry to bring us all together to fight – not just to protect the rights we've gained, but to keep pushing for the ones still out of reach. We all share a common goal, and we can only get there together. We've got to remember that lifting each other up is the aim, not dragging each other down in the service of a system that wants to divide and conquer us.

Bimbo isn't a memoir, but it does tell some stories from my life. This book is based on my own experiences and thoughts – thoughts which are always changing and evolving. If there are parts of it that you disagree with, *good*. It's important to acknowledge that there isn't one way to do womanhood. No one rule about how to be a feminist. We are all doing our best in a world of mixed messages and I, like everyone else, am full of contradictions. I want to be unflinchingly honest in these pages, and that means sharing all parts of myself, including my mistakes and imperfections. I am by no means a finished product. I'm still constantly unpicking and unlearning and even cringing at things I used to think or say. You may feel that way too, so I just want to mention that I'm not on any kind of pedestal either. I'm no feminist scholar with lots of letters after my name; I'm learning about feminism as I go. Instead, I am just a girl who was born confident, spent a chunk of my life losing that confidence, then the next part getting it back.

While I am focusing on living within a patriarchy – a society largely shaped by men, for men, which prioritises male needs, ambitions and desires at the expense of women – it's important to acknowledge that other systems also shape our experiences.

White supremacy, for example, operates through a racial hierarchy that affords white people better treatment and greater access to power. Capitalism is an economic system built on maximising profit, often for a few people at the expense of many. Class plays a huge role too, influencing not just the resources we have access to, but how seriously we're listened to, how we're judged, and how free we are to speak up. Nepotism grants access and opportunities to those with the right family connections. And many religious codes continue to privilege straight men and reinforce traditional gender roles.

Depending on the colour of your skin, the amount of

money you have, the schools you and your parents went to, your sexual orientation, or whether you identify as a man, a woman, or outside that binary, you're going to face greater or lesser challenges in life.

This book is written from my own lived experience as a white, cisgender woman navigating life in a patriarchal society. As such, much of my language is gendered, reflecting the realities I've personally faced and the systemic sexism that disproportionately affects women. But let me be clear: feminism is for everyone. The fight for gender equality must include men, trans women, non-binary people, and anyone whose identity challenges the rigid gender norms imposed by patriarchy. The same system that tells women to shrink also harms those who don't conform to traditional expectations of gender and sexuality. Our liberation is bound together. As a white woman, I know I have a responsibility to use my voice to support Black and brown women who face the compounded barriers of racism. Because if white women aren't bringing others with us in the fight for equality, what we're asking for isn't equality, it's privilege.

These themes are often dismissed today as simply being *woke,* but I would argue that is just another example of how those in power seek to divide us and maintain inequality. Unlike the weaponisation of the term 'woke', none of these ideas are new. Capitalism has been critiqued since the beginning of the industrial revolution; working-class movements and labour strikes have challenged class inequality for centuries; atheism gained traction in the late eighteenth century; white supremacy has been challenged since the beginning of the abolitionist movement; and the first wave of feminism started in *1848* with the first women's rights convention. Don't let anyone convince you that caring about inequality or injustice is fake news, or some kind of modern-day hysteria.

Over the years, my dismay and frustrations with the status quo have been transformational, and my rage has fuelled me to question why things are the way they are. I've become more curious about gender roles and the expectations that are placed on us from the moment we are born. I've desperately wanted to unravel why we so often accept the timelines, milestones, limitations and rules prescribed for women as if they were predestined, just because we were born female.

My rage isn't just about the collective experience of being a woman, but also the personal injustices so many of us face individually. The unfair double standards, the sexism, the hyper-sexualisation of our bodies, the uphill battle for equality. When I look back on a lot of what I went through in my girlhood, my adolescence and my early twenties, I feel a deep sadness for the child and young woman I once was. I also hold a lot of regret at how much I tolerated.

When I found myself single in my late twenties and early thirties, I became acutely aware of the imbalanced and frankly outdated pressures still placed on women. Instead of breaking me, that time lit a fire inside me. I began to realise that so many of the things that had stripped me of confidence were never my fault. And I hoped I could help other women and girls recognise how their experiences, drip by drip, had done the same.

Motherhood deepened my feminism in a way that surprised me. So much so that a good third of this book is about the discoveries I've made and the wild ride it has been. It was only once I became a mother myself – to a little boy called Alfie and a daughter called Ada – that I realised how much I had judged other mums, and how much of that came from internalised misogyny. That perspective has only strengthened my desire for change and understanding. Once I found my voice and confidence, I vowed never to be silent again.

No little girl is born a 'bimbo'. She doesn't arrive into the world as a 'prude', 'bitch' or 'slag' – nor any of the endless insults the English language has created to dismiss, reduce and disempower women.

In so many ways, I feel that I owe this book to my daughter. I owe it to all our daughters. And maybe our sons too.

So, let's begin.

Content warning:
This book contains descriptions of sexual assault, bullying, self-harm, body hatred and fat phobia, pregnancy and childbirth.

BIMBO
ˈbɪm.boʊ
noun

a derogatory term for a woman who is considered physically attractive but intellectually vapid. The implication that beauty and intelligence are mutually exclusive reduces a woman to her looks, positioning her as superficial, silly and sexually available.

The *bimbo* is typically portrayed as hyper-feminine, hyper-sexualised, and often infantilised. She's dismissed as a joke, a liability, or an object of lust. The term has long been weaponised to discredit, objectify and belittle women – especially those who embrace femininity or express their sexuality.

In recent years, some have begun to reclaim *bimbo* as a symbol of empowerment – celebrating femininity, self-expression, and subverting the idea that being hot and clever are mutually exclusive.

Bimbo. That's what they call me when they disagree with me on TV. Not 'misguided'. Not 'uninformed'. Just . . . *bimbo*. Because I have blonde hair and breasts and the audacity to talk about politics. Because I sit on a sofa in makeup and a dress and speak with conviction. Because I don't smile sweetly while I say it. It's not about my ideas, it's about my very existence. Because I am a woman stepping out of the box she was given. Still feminine, still visible, still loud. Very much 'too much'. It's criticism and vitriol that none of the men I work with will ever receive.

'Bimbo' comes from the Italian word for 'little boy' and used to be used to describe both men and women. However, by the 1980s and '90s, it had shifted to become a very specific insult aimed at women who were attractive, hyper-feminine, sexualised, and therefore assumed to be stupid. A woman in heels couldn't possibly be clever. A woman with cleavage couldn't possibly have an opinion worth hearing. A woman with lip gloss couldn't possibly be serious. Because fashion is femininity and femininity is frivolous. Like all the other derogatory terms we will explore in this book, *bimbo* is a convenient label. One designed to dismiss and discredit us. To pop our confidence like a balloon. It's especially weaponised when women step into male-dominated spaces – like politics, business or media – and dare to stay feminine while doing it. But maybe that's the point.

I used to say I wasn't into politics. I thought politics was something men in suits did in rooms with no windows. Something dry. Something far away. *BORING*, I'd think. But over time, I realised that everything that made me feel small, ashamed, silenced or unsafe was political.

Being slut-shamed as a teenager? Political. Because laws, education and media narratives shape how female sexuality is viewed and judged.

Being pitied for being single in my thirties? Political. Because marriage and motherhood are still protected and privileged by legal, financial and social systems, reinforcing that a woman's value is tied to being partnered.

Being judged for getting childcare and going back to work? Political. Because the cost of childcare, parental leave laws and the lack of recognition for unpaid domestic labour are all decided by government policy.

Knowing that if I ever reported rape, I'd be put on trial more than the man who hurt me? Political. Because the criminal justice system has abysmal conviction rates for sexual violence.

All the derogatory terms that have been targeted at me through my life were meant to shut me up and to undermine my confidence. To make me back away from the fight. But they have had the opposite effect. I started reading and then I started talking. And, now, I'm lucky enough to be a regular voice on one of the UK's most iconic daytime sofas. On *This Morning*, I have the chance to speak up about social justice, to call out inequality, and to hold the powerful to account. And when I do, the insults and threats come flooding in online.

Of course, people aren't always going to agree with me – and that's okay. My aim isn't to be *right* (in any sense of the word!) but to encourage people to consider a different perspective. We all come from different lives, backgrounds and circumstances, so of course we will see things differently at times. I'm learning and *un*learning daily, and my own opinions are always evolving. What I have come to realise is that my upbringing – and my journey from youth to midlife – is my superpower. I've mixed in different circles, I've lived in the north and the south, the city and the countryside. I understand the codes of farmers, but also the manners of aristocratic landowners. I know how the rich see the poor – and how the poor see the rich. I spent so long feeling like an outsider, but now I know that life was showing me it all, giving me insight into different communities and their attitudes, and helping me see the systems that lie above and below them all.

I have come to understand that politics isn't something we can shy away from. It's in our homes, our classrooms, our bank accounts and our bodies. Every policy passed affects women – our health, our choices, our safety, our livelihoods. And yet the spaces where those decisions are made are still overwhelmingly male. If we believe that politics isn't for women, we will continue to be the ones paying the price. In the UK Parliament, just 35 per cent of our representatives in the House of Commons and the House of Lords are women. We're still a minority in the very rooms where our futures are decided. And when women do make it into those rooms, the sexism doesn't stop, it shapeshifts.

So even if you find politics to be dull and totally dry, like I once did, I hope this book helps show why it matters. I hope it persuades you to engage, to question and to form your own opinions and viewpoints on some of the topics I cover on this rollercoaster ride that is existing in a female body in 2025.

So here I am. 'Girly'? Yep. 'Political'? Absolutely. Guess what? This 'bimbo' can do both.

GIRLHOOD

BOSSY
ˈbɒs.i
adjective

a word used to criticise someone, usually a girl or woman, for being assertive or taking charge. It implies overstepping or showing an undesirable level of authority and is often used to shame girls for showing leadership or confidence. A gendered reprimand that teaches girls early on that power and likeability cannot coexist, reinforcing the idea that women should be passive, agreeable and deferential.

Male equivalent: *Assertive, confident, a leader*
Note that none of these equivalent words are insults – there is no widely used male equivalent that carries the same critical, belittling tone. When boys and men show the exact same behaviours, they are usually praised or rewarded.

1.
Princess

Have you ever thought about how strange it is that, from the moment we're born, there are already expectations placed on who we can be – all depending on whether we're born a boy or a girl? Before we can even understand words, we're wrapped in pink or blue, handed princesses or dinosaurs, and praised for being pretty or strong. We're taught which colours are 'appropriate', what clothes to wear, and what toys to play with – all before we're remotely able to choose them for ourselves. And the rules are clear: pink for girls, blue for boys. Even if you don't follow these rules yourself, you'll be aware of them.

I was born in a hospital in the Northumbrian town of Hexham on an ordinary Thursday in 1987. That was the moment my parents found out they were having a little girl. By the time I had my own children thirty-four years later, things had changed – it had become far more common to know your baby's sex before the birth, thanks to ultrasound scans and advanced testing. These days, many people throw gender reveal parties with balloons, cakes and coloured smoke. I celebrated each of my babies with confetti cannons: blue for my boy Alfie, pink for my girl Ada.

When I was born, my parents' friends joked they'd need to lock me up because I'd be trouble. After leaving hospital as a baby, I came home to the dairy farm where I grew up and

I wore dresses and played with toys marketed for girls. Our family was fairly traditional – my dad was a farmer who drove tractors and took on the more 'masculine' roles, i.e. mowing the lawn, fixing things. He's still the handiest person I know. My mum, despite working full-time as a hairdresser, was mostly responsible for the domestic duties and raising us.

Growing up on a farm gave me a very specific kind of childhood. Apparently, I once went around collecting dead rabbits and hugging each one, assuring them that 'God would look after them in heaven.' Another time, my mum came home to find dead moles propped up in the garden – I'd tried to save them by sitting them upright in their holes.

But when I wasn't scooping up dead animals, I was playing with dolls, my Wendy house, and my toy kitchen. My favourites were always my Barbies. Mum once told me I came downstairs for dinner in a rush, explaining I had to be quick because I'd left Ken alone with all the Barbies and he wasn't to be trusted. Clearly, I had an early understanding of sexual dynamics . . . While I pushed my toy pushchair, my older brother played with cars, tractors, dinosaurs and Teenage Mutant Ninja Turtles.

Back then, I loved being called a princess. It felt like the highest compliment, and I was totally obsessed with the idea of being one. Mum once told me she'd heard me rustling around my room after bedtime for several nights in a row. One evening, curiosity got the better of her, and she came in to check. She found me fast asleep under my duvet, fully dressed in my princess costume. When she asked why, I replied, 'I can't go to the ball in my pyjamas. The prince won't pick me.' Tell me you watched too many Disney films without telling me you watched too many Disney films . . .

When I wasn't dressed as a princess, I wore pastel-coloured

dresses, skirts and tops. Looking back, some of the outfits were peak '90s: lime-green dresses with oversized black polka dots, worn with matching giant ribbons. My brother dressed up as superheroes and wore classic 'boy' clothes.

By the time I started school, I had a very clear idea of what it meant to be a girl – and what it meant to be a boy. Of course, I don't remember those early years in detail, so I didn't feel the social conditioning tightening around me. I didn't yet understand how certain behaviours are encouraged while others are quietly discouraged. As a child, I simply absorbed it all. It's only now, with the benefit of hindsight, that I can see those moments for what they really were: tiny but powerful nudges that shaped how I saw myself. Nudges away from self-worth, away from confidence, away from who I might have been if I'd been allowed to choose freely.

I didn't question any of it – not until I had children of my own.

2.
Like a Girl

Having children of your own really makes you reflect on the way in which you were raised, and how the messages you were taught shaped you. But it also forces you to question the world in which you're raising your own children, and the beliefs being instilled in them.

I noticed how the world treated my kids differently from the moment they were born. Well-meaning friends and family joked that Alfie would be a 'heartbreaker'. I hope not, I thought. By this point, I'd been on the receiving end of heartbreak from several awful men and hoped Alfie would grow up with much more respect for people's hearts and minds. When Ada was born, she was met with the same public commentary I had been – jokes about needing to 'lock her up'. My partner Tommy even joked she wouldn't be allowed to date until she was thirty. 'Yes, she will,' I replied.

It made me realise how strange it is that we joke about locking up baby girls to protect them from boys. How strange our world is, where we're comfortable objectifying and projecting messed-up social standards onto infants? These descriptions might sound harmless – even affectionate – but they're early lessons in gender roles. What they actually teach is that boys can't be expected to control themselves around attractive girls, and that girls must be kept out of reach to protect them from male violence. That girls must be policed to avoid bringing shame on the family. That boys who are handsome will inevitably cause pain. When you boil it down, it's all pretty grim – especially considering we're talking about babies.

And this is where victim-blaming starts. These throw-away remarks teach us that it's a girl's job to limit her freedom to accommodate male behaviour. That it's her fault if *something happens*, because she should have stayed safely indoors. To the dads who say their daughters won't be allowed to date until they're mature adults, I always want to ask – why? Who are you afraid they'll encounter? Men? If so, why don't we ever say we'll lock up our sons? The seeds planted by these comments grow into the belief that it's women and girls who must change, shrink or hide – rather than expecting boys and men to be better. That's a terrifying principle to grow up with.

Even the compliments differ. Alf is praised for being funny or clever. With Ada, it's almost always that she's beautiful. Of course, we're allowed to coo over babies if that's our natural response – and she *is* beautiful. But when was the last time you complimented a little girl, or her parents, on something other than her looks? I catch myself doing it too, because that's how we're conditioned to view female value, but I'm constantly correcting my own language. If a child is always praised first for being pretty or cute, it sends the message that looks are what matter most. In a world so obsessed with image, it's not a stretch for a child to start believing that being attractive is more valuable than being clever, kind, funny or capable. These messages shape our children's sense of themselves, and not in good ways.

Another common compliment Ada receives is being called 'a little princess'. I once laughed when my mum came down to visit and declared, 'Who's a little princess?' and Alf proudly said, 'Me!' He's unknowingly breaking down gender norms one comment at a time. I never call Ada a princess. Despite growing up obsessed with them myself, adulthood showed me how unrealistic and limiting the fantasy of being 'picked' can be. I don't understand why we still push that fantasy. Especially when we've seen what happens to our real-life princesses, like Diana or Meghan, or even Kate. The role is still defined by the man you marry. Do I want my daughter aspiring to be someone's prize? Or do I want her to dream bigger? She can love dressing up as princesses if she chooses to, in the same way that Alfie can, but I won't push it on her.

Through following my children's interests, I've come to learn how many of the 'traditions' I took as biological inevitabilities are actually just learned behaviours. We grow up thinking boys like boy things and girls like girl things, but most of it has nothing to do with biology.

Take pink and blue. If you ask Alfie his favourite colours, he will proudly tell you that it is 'pink, purple, rainbows, golden sparkle and glitter'. Who can blame him – they are *great* colours! But I'm sure many would say they are 'girly' colours. Did you know that, as recently as 1918, pink was actually recommended for boys and blue for girls? Earnshaw's Infants' Department wrote: 'The generally accepted rule is pink for the boys and blue for the girls. The reason is that pink, being a more decided and stronger colour, is more suitable for the boy, while blue, which is more delicate and daintier, is prettier for the girl.'

It wasn't until after the Second World War that pink-for-girls and blue-for-boys began to stick, thanks largely to marketing. Then, during the women's liberation movement of the 1960s and '70s, second-wave feminists pushed back against gendered conditioning, and pink fell out of fashion entirely.

There were two years in the 1970s when Sears, the American chain of department stores, didn't feature a single item of pink toddler clothing. But by the 1980s – with the conservative backlash and the rise of ultrasound scans – pink made a roaring comeback.

Walk into any children's clothing shop today and the gendered colours hit you straight away. Boys get blue, green, and slogans like 'Future Leader', 'Adventure Awaits' and 'Boss'. Girls get pink, pastels, and messaging like 'Pretty', 'Princess' or 'Little Cutie'. Even the animals are gendered. Boys are targeted with sharks, lions and dinosaurs – apex predators. Girls are served bunnies, butterflies and deer – gentle, vulnerable prey. Once you see it, you can't unsee it. Boys' clothes are practical, durable, and made for movement. Girls' clothes? Delicate, restrictive, and weirdly revealing. I've lost count of how many times I've gone to buy Ada a pair of shorts only to find they barely cover her nappy. Even toddler girls' clothes are shaped by adult ideas of female presentation. I love dresses, but Ada mostly wears trousers unless it's a special occasion, because so many girls' clothes are just so impractical. At the park, skirts and dresses trip her up and stop her being able to climb. It's clear that boys' clothes are made for exploring the world. Girls' clothes are made for sitting still and looking cute.

One moment that really forced me to question this gendered dressing was a couple of years ago when I shot a magazine cover with both Alfie and Ada. We had a stylist sorting the outfits, as is typical for shoots, and, on the day, Ada and I were dressed in beautiful dresses, while Alf was put in shorts and a T-shirt. He got really upset. He couldn't understand why we got to wear the pretty clothes, and he didn't. He insisted on wearing a dress, but there wasn't one in his size. I text Tommy and asked him to pick one up on his way home and he came back with an Elsa dress. Alf beamed. 'I'm just like Mummy,' he said. For him, wearing the dress was about love and admiration for me. And I wondered, why don't we allow boys to look up to women?

That admiration shows up in toys too. Like many other boys, Alf has always loved dolls. They help him explore relationships, emotions, and care through play. I've noticed that some parents — and especially, from my experience, fathers — push back on boys playing with 'girly' toys. I often look at my partner pushing our kids in the pram and wonder how we ever convinced ourselves that dolls and prams are only for girls. It still blows my mind that roleplaying caregiving is so widely accepted as 'girly'. Men also care for children — it's called fatherhood. Playing with dolls fosters empathy, creativity and social skills — qualities that benefit all children, regardless of gender. Why wouldn't we want boys to be nurturing too? What could be more masculine than modelling what it means to be a good father?

Much like the colour divide, the strong gender split in toy marketing is a fairly modern invention. With the rise of mass production and booming consumer culture after the Second World War, gendered toy marketing ramped up. The 1950s and '60s saw a surge in ads reinforcing traditional gender roles: pink kitchen sets for girls, action figures and cars for boys. Despite feminist pushback, by the 1980s the divide held strong, and still does today.

Why do we tell boys they can't wear dresses, play with dolls or paint their nails? Is it deep-rooted homophobia? That fear some parents have that, if their son is 'feminine', he might be gay? And so what if he is? Painting your nails isn't the same as sexuality — it's just curiosity. But even if our children are gay, or trans, or non-binary, the last thing we should do is shame them for it. We can't shame a child into being more masculine or feminine, any more than we can change who they are. And this isn't just about protecting our own kids — it's also about helping them not become the ones who unknowingly bully others for being different. Because when we have rigid norms, anyone who dares to step out of them is bullied back into line using labels. And it harms both boys and girls.

Gender norms teach children which parts of themselves — and each other — are acceptable, and which are not. Alf is only four and he's already come home with comments like 'only girls do their hair'. I had to point out that my hair stylist, Michael, is a man. It shows how early these ideas take hold. Gender norms aren't just about clothes and colours — they're social blueprints. And while none of us get it right all the time (least of all me), just being aware of what we say and do can help us raise children who feel safe being themselves.

When we police our children's interests, traits or clothes based on their gender, we don't just shape who they think they're allowed to be — we shape who they think they're allowed to value, admire and respect. We subtly teach them that 'girly' means 'less than'. And those lessons don't stay in childhood. They follow us into adulthood. It all starts here: with pink and blue. If we don't question it, we raise children who begin from their earliest days to shrink themselves — and shrink each other too.

3.
Bossy Boots

Before I even started school, I had already absorbed so many messages about what was appropriate for girls and what was exclusively for boys. But it was at school that I began to learn how labels are used to keep us in line.

I have fond memories of primary school: I remember all my teachers' names, and I remember sitting in the main hall for assembly. I even remember singing 'Morning Has Broken' at the top of my lungs while competing with another little girl called Deborah to see who could sing the loudest. I can still recall us locking eyes with each other, determined to out-sing the other.

Whether that kind of competitiveness or desire to stand out is something you see as a positive sign of confidence or not, what was abundantly clear was that adults were on a mission to stamp the volume out of me. As a five- or six-year-old, what stuck with me most was the injustice of being constantly told off for being *bossy*. Whether it was by my teachers, my mum, or someone else's mum at a party or in the playground, it was always the same. I might have been organising a game of 'mams and dads', telling other kids off for talking in class, or getting everyone to sit in a circle at my birthday party so we could play Pass the Parcel. No matter the intention, I learned very early on that everyone – especially the adults – wanted me to pipe down.

No one saw it as an early sign of leadership or confidence. No one said these were skills I might need as a woman. Instead, it was hammered into me that being 'bossy' would make people hate me. That I'd be seen as controlling. That it wasn't appropriate for a little girl. As an adult, I look back and feel both sorrow and envy for little me. I spent so much of my adulthood trying to find my voice and my boundaries, and there I was, confidently setting them as a child, only to have them squashed out of me.

What frustrates me most about the word *bossy* is that it's almost exclusively used to describe girls. My daughter has often been called bossy, and even when it's said affectionately, I always make the point that this kind of assertiveness is something that will serve her well in life. I hope she's always bossy! When a little boy behaves the same way, people nudge each other and say he's a CEO in the making. But for Ada? She's already being told to change her tune.

I'd love to say that *bossy* was the only criticism adults threw my way, but it wasn't. I was also endlessly told off for being *too loud*—

'Ashley, the whole school doesn't need to hear your opinions. Keep your voice to yourself.'

And *too opinionated*—

'Ashley, boys don't like girls with such big views.'

What those adults were really saying was: *You are too much.*

When we teach girls to stay quiet, to avoid taking up space, and to prioritise being agreeable over being authentic, they internalise it. A young girl who stands up for herself is often labelled *difficult*. A boy doing the same is admired for his boldness.

Over time, those repeated messages push girls to believe their voices are less important. That they're better off in the background. That being bossy, loud or opinionated will isolate them socially.

And yet, considering the world we're sending them out into, the *last* thing we should be doing is teaching our girls to swallow their thoughts and make themselves small.

Dealing with a spirited, high-volume child isn't always easy. But encouraging their natural confidence will serve them well for life.

These early lessons teach girls to doubt their worth and potential. They learn to diminish themselves to fit with societal expectations, prioritising being liked over being respected. And these harmful foundations don't just disappear with age. They can manifest in women's struggles daily, whether it's asserting themselves at work, negotiating their salaries, or saying *no* without guilt – both personally and professionally. The problem often isn't in the behaviour of girls, it's in how deeply embedded these messages are in our culture.

We have to stand up to these harmful norms. Adults need to recognise the power of their words and actions and make sure they're not reinforcing stereotypes that limit girls' potential. Encouraging girls to speak up, take risks and embrace leadership roles is a start. And if we want them to lead? We need to stop calling them 'bossy'.

4.
Fitting In

Up until this point, I feel like I had an ordinary and happy childhood. The choice that changed my life forever was when my parents decided to send me to boarding school, aged nine. It was a very unusual decision. Until my brother started three years before me, no one in my family had ever gone to private school or even sixth form, so the concept was completely alien to everyone. My parents were hardworking people who made enormous compromises to give me so many opportunities and privileges, for which I will always be incredibly grateful. But, in retrospect, this was the moment I went from being a happy-go-lucky child to becoming self-conscious. It was the first time I felt aware that I didn't quite fit in, either at school or at home.

In the UK, only 6 per cent of kids are educated privately[1] and only 0.7 per cent of those children board.[2] What we know is that children who attend fee-paying schools have access to a host of privileges that many state school kids simply don't. The private/state divide has long been argued to be one of the roots of social inequality in this country. Clumping the wealthiest, and often most powerful, families together in schools with very little economic diversity creates a distinct and highly skewed environment for children to grow up in. It also offers the privately educated enormous advantages through networking. There's a reason that, out of Britain's fifty-eight Prime Ministers, twenty went to the same school: Eton. Just eleven have been state educated.

In the UK, the roots of this privilege can run centuries deep and they have created what's been described as a sophisticated form of social segregation. *'Which school did you go to?'* is still a question that can open or close doors. Yet for all their advantages, boarding schools – many of which involve sending children away from their parents as young as seven – can also come with complicated emotional consequences. Psychologists have even coined a term for it: *boarding school syndrome* – the long-term effects of which can include emotional detachment, difficulty forming relationships, and low self-esteem. Sounds about right. In recent years, several boarders, including aristocrat Charles Spencer, have written about their harrowing experiences at boarding schools in the '70s, lifting the lid on the profound horror and abuse many endured.

I mention all this not just to highlight how unusual it was that I ended up in one of these elite schools, but also to offer context about the culture – a culture that has a disproportionate impact, because so many of our leaders and decision-makers were raised within these institutions. If we want to understand many of society's attitudes to class, gender or race, we need to look at where those in power first learned their values. Often, it's in the halls of schools like these.

I can still remember dropping my brother off for the first time, sitting in the back seat of the car, mesmerised by the grandeur of his new school. It was set on a country estate about forty-five minutes from our home, with a huge, sweeping driveway. The school building itself looked like something out of a period drama. I was completely obsessed. I loved the uniform. I loved the sport. I loved how much attention the teachers would give me. I was dead set on going. I say it was my parents' decision to pack me off to school, but my older brother had been offered a scholarship and I'd found it *terribly* unfair that he got to go, and I didn't; I begged them to let me go too. '*I want to go to boarding school. Why does Stuart get to go, and I don't?*' (Even without the school, I'd clearly already nailed the entitlement part.)

My dad had left school at sixteen without O-levels, and my mum left at sixteen too. Both had felt they had no choice. They were expected to work on the family farms they'd grown up on, so had limited experience of the education system. Both of them were determined to prioritise our education to give us access to opportunities they hadn't been able to access themselves. After they agreed to let me go on a trial overnight stay, I was officially sold on it, and I ended up getting a scholarship, just like my brother. What I didn't know as a child was the financial burden this placed on my family, despite the scholarship. I had no idea that my Gran had had to contribute to make it happen. And I don't think any of us realised how much I would be leaving behind the world as we knew it.

Even though I'd used all the negotiation skills of a determined seven-year-old, my mum recently told me that my dad always stood firm when people around him had said, '*At least you only have to think about your lad – the two girls can go to the local.*' I know they were excited about the opportunities a private education could offer both boys and girls. Despite their traditional outlook, they never wanted me to be dependent on a man.

However, what they hadn't really accounted for was that they were sending us straight into the lion's den of the British class system. By the time I came home for the first break, I already felt like part of a different world – not quite feeling like I belonged to either. In some ways, I feel like my parents sent their children off to school . . . and we never really came back.

Before going to boarding school, I'd never really considered class. At my local state school, everyone came from more or less the same background and sounded the same. To my knowledge, all the parents worked hard in retail or beauty, hospitality, farming, or other forms of manual labour and trades. No one worked for a big corporate company or held what some might consider 'high-flying' professional roles. It was a big talking point if someone's niece or nephew had moved to a city and got a 'fancy' job in an office.

But from the moment I put on my uniform and waved goodbye to my parents, I became acutely aware of my position in the class pecking order. (Spoiler alert: it wasn't exactly at the top.) Just before I started boarding school, my parents sold the family farm and bought a Bed & Breakfast in the same area. I can only imagine what a big step it was for my dad to walk away from his farm, which had been his father's before him – especially with no other work experience. We moved into one of the biggest houses in town. It had twelve bedrooms, a big garden with three separate levels, and even a field. The thing that blew my mind most was the fact that we'd inherited a four-poster bed in one of the rooms. It looked like something a Disney princess would sleep in. *We must be royalty now*, I thought. I even went to school and told everyone about it – except I told everyone it was a 'three-poster bed'. I suppose, by that point, I had started to develop some idea of what material wealth meant.

But starting boarding school introduced me to wealth – and social position – on a whole new level. For starters, I was one of the only girls in my year without a title. These ranged from Lady to The Honourable. Three of the girls lived in *actual* castles. I learned that it was 'chavvy' if your house had a door number – a thought I still laugh at every day when I walk through the door of my London terrace. Every Sunday after church, we had to write a good old-fashioned letter home, and I would watch as my classmates addressed theirs to the Duke and Duchess, or to various Lords and Ladies. My parents still have countless letters I wrote to them with fake titles at the top – all because I wanted so badly to fit in. Who would have thought that plain old *Mr and Mrs* was something a nine-year-old could learn to be embarrassed about?

Let me just stress here that, despite the class differences I'm about to describe, I absolutely *loved* the prep school where I boarded from nine until twelve. When I talk about teasing, it really was just that – not bullying. The teachers were exceptional, and the headmaster made a point of reassuring me and my parents that we were welcome at the school. I acknowledge the privilege, the sacrifice, and the amazing memories I made. But I'd be lying if I said it didn't also leave a mark. The teasing might have been mild, but the messages stuck. The quiet signals about where I sat in the class hierarchy. Today we might call them microaggressions, but back then it just felt like a long list of reasons why I didn't entirely belong. As much as there were so many positive things to take away, that doesn't mean that time didn't have a lasting impact on my confidence.

At school, I was considered poor. Working-class. The first thing I was teased about was my accent. I arrived at school with a strong Geordie voice. I pronounced my 'a' like the vowel in *cat*, not the long 'ar' sound expected in Southern accents. If I wanted a bath, I'd ask for a *b-a-th*, not a *b-ar-th*.

Once, a group of boys ran up to me saying, '*Have you heard the new Geordie girl? Go on, say something!*'

'*What d'ya want us to say?*' I asked.

'Oh my God, hilarious. Do the "a" again – the "a" is HILAAARIOUS!'

They once asked me to spell *geography*, then stopped me when I got to the 'o', and made me repeat it again and again as they laughed. I felt like a performing monkey. A *northern* monkey.

After a couple of weeks of being singled out, I decided to fake my accent to be more like them. But no one tells you that having a 'posh' accent isn't as straightforward as replacing one vowel with another. When I asked my friend where my *hat* was, I still remember her confused expression as she pointed at my chest. She thought I was asking about my *heart*. Being posh was tricky.

The first time I went home and saw one of my friends, she pulled me up on my accent straight away: *'Why ya talkin' like that for? D'ya think you're better than uz now?'* And she wasn't the only one. Pretty much everyone commented – kids, adults, even my own family. I still remember my dad looking particularly embarrassed once in the supermarket when he bumped into his friends. At school, I sounded too regional. At home, I sounded too posh.

For a nine-year-old, this feeling of not belonging anywhere was too complicated to understand. But it stayed with me for such a long time. Even into adulthood.

I felt a bit like Ariel in *The Little Mermaid*. She wanted legs to be worthy of Eric, I wanted a posh accent to be worthy of my peers. I suppose both of us had to trade in our voice for acceptance.

To this day, I still speak with neat, sharp vowels, but my accent became one of my biggest insecurities. It has driven so many assumptions about who I am. It's made me feel like a fraud. Like I'd betrayed my family and my roots. Like I might be found out. And I also hate the assumption that I've been born with a silver spoon in my mouth. Bias against regional accents — or accents full stop — hasn't gone anywhere. In fact, a recent study showed that around a quarter of people have been mocked or criticised for their accent in the workplace.[3]

Of course, it wasn't just my accent that made me stand out. In fact, there were countless times where I was hyper aware of my very different background at school. And, unfortunately, I couldn't just change the way I said my 'a' to fit in. There were several times when my dad would drop me off at school in the wagon before heading to work — he became a truck driver for a while as a way to earn more money. I'm sure you don't need to be that familiar with boarding school culture to know that I'm probably the only person in its history, other than maybe my siblings, to have ever been dropped off in a lorry. Today, I can appreciate how hard that must have been for my parents. Not only the financial pressure, but the time pressure too. Both working two jobs to make ends meet, and likely feeling judged by the other parents. But at the time? I was just embarrassed.

Why couldn't my parents just be normal?

Just after I turned eleven, I was lucky enough to spend some time in school in France. Our boarding school co-owned a chateau there — of course it did. To this day, it remains one of the best experiences of my life, and it inspired me to study French all the way through to university level.

If boarding school took me out of my hometown, going to school in France opened my eyes to a whole new universe. The chateau was co-owned by another British prep school down south, and what I quickly learned was that southern British posh is a different level to northern British posh.

Before I went away, my mum decided to give me a new haircut — that was her job, after all. Looking back, I'm certain she tried to make me look as undesirable as possible by giving me some pretty wild styles, especially as I entered my teenage years! But, on this occasion, she went with the Victoria Beckham bob, affectionately known as the 'POB'. For those unfamiliar, the POB involved longer pieces at the front and very short hair at the back. It was bang on trend at the time.

What I learned very quickly was that posh people don't *do* fashion trends. Especially not ones inspired by a WAG. My new nickname became 'Fashion Witch', and I was teased about that haircut for the entire term.

It wasn't just the kids. I'll never forget one particular teacher at my secondary school. He was a parody of the elitist, chauvinistic southerner that gives everyone below the Watford Gap a bad name. For whatever reason, he loved to put me in my place. One lunchtime, I must've said something a little too 'uppity' for his liking, and in front of everyone at the table he said, *'Your dad's obviously into football because, like other northern men, he's probably unemployed and has nothing better to do.'*

I took real childish pleasure in reminding him that my dad paid his wages. These are just a few of the many moments where I navigated being *othered*. Teased for being different. And I really, really wanted to fit in. In retrospect, I think the problem was that no one ever sat me down – at home or school – to give me any kind of warning that I might be treated differently to the other little kids in their little uniforms. Nobody ever empowered me to be proud of my background or gave me the tools or words to know how to respond. I've never forgotten those barbs, because they pierced me so deeply. Over time, they made me believe there were parts of me, because of who my parents were (or weren't), that I should hide. These insecurities overwhelmed me as a young person.

It didn't help that back home I had similar experiences, but in the opposite direction. I can understand how disorienting it must have felt for my parents, but they were often so defensive about my new habits and manners. They'd laugh at how I spoke, and any time I said or did something that was completely normal at school but unfamiliar to them, they'd defensively say, '*Do you think that's normal?*'

Which 'normal' was I meant to follow? The normal at home or the normal at school?

This conundrum had a catastrophic impact on my sense of self and identity. Most people assume they are 'normal' growing up, as I had before I went to boarding school. But, now, I felt like I had to work really hard not to be *abnormal*. I felt like being me was never enough.

I carried shame about my background for most of my teens and twenties. As an adult, it took me a long time to walk into a room without assuming people disliked me. I always felt self-conscious, like I was saying or doing the wrong thing. Now that I'm on the other side, and while I deeply recognise my privileges in life, I have enormous empathy for anyone who doesn't feel like they fit in a space because of who they are or where they come from. I'm not sure I'll ever have a true sense of belonging anywhere – that deep feeling of being *home* or knowing what *normal* is. What I do know is that I am proud of being northern, I'm proud of my parents for everything they did for me and my siblings, and I'm proud of little me for trying to straddle two normal-but-abnormal worlds.

TART

tɑːt

noun

a derogatory term for a woman perceived as sexually provocative, flirtatious, or dressed in a way deemed 'inappropriate' or 'cheap'. Often used to shame women for their clothing, behaviour or sexual expression. It carries a strong classist undertone that implies bad taste, low status and promiscuity.

Male equivalent: While men can be called terms like lad, player or stud for similar behaviour, these words tend to reward sexual confidence rather than punish it. There's no true male equivalent to tart because men are rarely shamed for the same reasons. Tart reflects a culture that polices female sexuality and uses language to keep women modest, ashamed and controllable. It reinforces the double standard that a sexually confident man is successful, while a sexually confident woman is disgraceful.

5.
'Tarty-Warty Ashley'

Have you ever considered how many derogatory words aimed at women are focused on our sexual behaviour?

I was just eleven years old when the first sexualised insult was thrown my way. It happened shortly after getting my first bras. My mum had bought me two: a white one and a black one. I wore the black one most and felt really grown up, just like a lot of little girls taking their first steps into womanhood.

One day at school, I was wearing a tank top and, unbeknownst to me, my black bra straps were showing. Out of nowhere, one of my girlfriends turned to me and shouted, *'Ooo, TARTY-WARTY ASHLEY!'* loud enough for everyone to hear. Apparently, posh girls didn't wear black bras. Or at least they didn't show off their straps in public. I was mortified and the comment stuck with me for years. I didn't wear a black bra again for a long time.

For all the complicated experiences I had at school, I loved all the games we played in our free time. One of our favourites was named after the '90s cartoon *The Poddington Peas*, where we'd wrap ourselves in duvets, jump at each other, and try to knock everyone down. But not all the games were quite so light-hearted.

The sexualisation of play at my school started on day one when I was just nine years old. The moment I stepped foot into the Common Room, which was the communal space where we all hung out, I was immediately confronted by two boys in the year above me. They told me they wouldn't let me out unless I snogged one of them. To be clear, they weren't looking for a peck, they wanted a full-on adult snog.

I said I didn't want to, but they were adamant they wouldn't let me out of the room until I did it. I was scared and wanted to get out of the room and the situation, so I did it. Or, more accurately, I let him do it. I still remember his name clearly. There was another incident with him a few years later.

At the time, we were having a party in the school pool, which in retrospect is quite unusual. One of the games involved lining up and pushing whoever we didn't fancy into the water. First all the girls lined up, then the boys. When I got pushed into the water, that same boy who'd coerced me into kissing him came over and started to repeatedly dunk me. I frantically looked around to see if anyone could help me as he laughed hysterically at my panic. The moment I caught my breath I'd be back underwater again. It felt like it went on forever. I don't remember how it stopped, but eventually it did. I was sobbing in fear. He said that we'd all been having fun, and I shouldn't be so sensitive. I never told anyone.

From as young as nine, we would play Spin the Pencil. The boys and girls would get together, sit in a circle, and quite literally spin a pencil. Whoever it landed on, you had to full-on snog – in front of everyone. We were so young that we didn't see it as anything sexual, it was just a game that we usually played in our year groups. We found it funny. These days, though, I often wonder who introduced it into the school and how it got passed down. Had one kid watched an older sibling playing Spin the Bottle perhaps? Who knows. But it does make me sad to think that we were all playing along as if it was the most normal thing in the world, which is a good example of how skewed a child's idea of 'normal' can get. I don't think the teachers knew about it, or at least, if they did, they never stopped it.

When we did finally receive a bit of sex education at the age of eleven, not only had we been snogging for years, but that guidance didn't even mention snogging, or consent, or what to do if we were locked in a common room by an older boy. We were simply taught about how babies are made, so I hardly connected the dots between that and the sexualised games I'd been playing for years. While I know that sex education has improved a lot and consent is now discussed in the classroom, it doesn't enter the curriculum until Year 4, when children are aged eight to nine. Given that 10 per cent of nine-year-olds are thought to have already seen pornography,[4] I think it's fair to say that schools still have a long way to go to empower and protect children.

6.
Aunt Flo

At school there was a hierarchical system of Matrons, or Matey, as we called them. Matrons were the women responsible for the domestic and medical arrangements at boarding school.

The hierarchy went like this:
Matey Min
Matey Mo
Matey Ma

Matey Min handled minor issues, such as putting us to bed or telling us off for making too much noise after lights out. Matey Ma was for major incidents – sickness, bad behaviour, or death.

The day I saw blood in my knickers, I decided it was definitely an incident for Matey Ma. Was there anything more MAJOR than bleeding from your bum?

I walked down the corridor and knocked on her private door, something I'd never done before. I still remember her face when she opened it and looked down at me. I told her I was dying. 'I'm bleeding,' I said. The moment she realised *where* I was bleeding from – an orifice I didn't even know existed – she smiled and said, 'Oh wonderful! Go and get the girls and bring them straight back!'

Ten minutes later, the girls in my year and I were sitting in Matey Ma's private room having a tea party to be educated about the menstrual cycle. She didn't produce pads, just tampons, and explained that there was, in fact, a third hole on our bodies – 'between the wee and the poo hole'. I was stunned. A THIRD HOLE? WHERE? WHY? HOW?

I went straight to the toilet with my friend Lucie to investigate. She also helped me to insert said tampon. Teamwork makes the dream work! That was really the only time I ever discussed periods with an adult. Sure, I had to ask my mum for tampons during the school holidays, but, beyond that, we never had a conversation about it. It felt shameful and embarrassing, especially because it had happened to me *before* everyone else. Best to just do it all in secret.

There was NOTHING more humiliating than asking your parents for tampons. Or, as I got older, having to run into the Spar near school and buy some, knowing a boy might walk in at any second and catch you buying these highly embarrassing, highly taboo products. Despite the fact that menstruation is a natural biological process, periods are still surrounded by stigma, secrecy and shame all over the world. This taboo is rooted in a mix of religious and cultural ideas that suggest periods are dirty or disgusting. Lots of women, even as adults, who know in theory that there's nothing dirty or embarrassing about periods, still hide their tampons when going to the loo. The shame doesn't just disappear as we mature.

Just like our 'girls-only' tea party, boys are usually left out of conversations about periods. That silence makes it feel secretive. We even see it in period product adverts, where blue liquid replaces red blood, reinforcing the idea that periods are too disgusting to be shown honestly. I once saw a meme that said, if men had periods, they'd wear tampons behind their ears like pencils. How many of us remember starting our period and having to smuggle a tampon up our sleeve to get to the toilet undetected?

Women and girls shouldn't have to hide period products – not in public, and not at home. Seeing tampons or pads in the bathroom should be as normal as seeing toothpaste.

I also wish my parents and school had made period products easily accessible, so I didn't always have to ask for them. It's up to us to challenge society's weirdness around periods. Kids will inevitably hear negative comments, whether from family, classmates, or even on TV, but we can talk openly about what they hear and we can correct it.

We can teach them that periods are a sign of a healthy body. That there is nothing dirty or shameful about them. This actually stumped me recently when I was on my period and using a pad. Alf followed me into the bathroom and looked at it in horror. His first question was why I was wearing a nappy. Then he asked why it was red.

I froze. I didn't know what to say.

Later, I looked up some age-appropriate responses:

- **Toddlers and young children**: 'It's something that happens to most women and girls when they grow up. It's normal and not scary.'
- **Primary school children**: 'Periods happen because the body is getting ready for a possible baby. If there's no baby, the body releases a little blood, and that's totally normal.'

We also need to use biological and factual language. When we rely on euphemisms like 'time of the month' or 'Aunt Flo', we reinforce the idea that periods are shameful or secret. We don't call breathing 'Puffy Uncle' or digestion 'Difficult Dad'.

Uterus. Menstruation. Period. Ovaries. Fallopian tubes. Womb lining. Bloody. Vagina. Vulva. Clitoris.

None of these are swear words – but many of us feel like that using them.

To stop this cycle, we can empower our children by showing them the range of options – so they're not trying to locate a mysterious third hole with a Tampax mini when period pants might have been a better option.

Understanding how the mechanics of our cycle work might also do wonders – we have different phases, for example: luteal, follicular, menstrual, ovulation – and help us connect the dots. It can explain why we feel amazing some days and flatlining on others. Why we might be smashing it at the gym one week and crying in the toilet the next. Why our confidence fluctuates. Why imposter syndrome feels louder some weeks than others. I'm spelling it out because it took me so long to realise that I wasn't depressed every month – I was just in my luteal phase. My confidence was being rocked by my hormones. So, what can we do to change the narrative? First, we need to teach all children about periods in an open, age-appropriate and factual way. Second, we need to include boys in the conversation. Not only will this help them understand what periods are, it might help girls feel less ashamed.

Armed with this knowledge, men would be able to support us far more compassionately – as partners, fathers, brothers, friends, colleagues. We deserve periods to be reframed by society. Because they are the reason every single person on this earth exists. You don't get much more powerful than that.

MAIDENHOOD

PICK-ME GIRL
pɪk mi gɜːl
noun

a woman or girl who seeks validation from men by putting down other women or aligning herself with male preferences, often by claiming to be 'not like other girls'. The term is usually used to mock women who appear to reject traits considered stereotypically feminine in order to appeal to the male gaze or gain social acceptance in male-dominated spaces.

Pick-Me Girl functions both as a critique of internalised misogyny and as a way women police each other's behaviour. While some use it to call out performative patriarchy, it can also silence women navigating a sexist world by doing what they feel they must to be accepted. Like many gendered terms, it exposes the impossible tightrope women must walk between being 'one of the girls' and being desirable to men.

Male equivalent: *Simp*
There's no widely used male counterpart that carries the same shaming or social policing function, as while simp is sometimes used to ridicule men who are overly attentive to women, it stems from a different cultural dynamic – punishing men for showing respect or admiration for women.

7.
'Not Like the Other Girls'

There isn't one clear age when we move from girlhood into womanhood, but I definitely noticed a shift after I got my period and moved to secondary school. I was sent to an all-girls boarding school most famous for having once educated the Brontë sisters: Maria, Elizabeth, Charlotte and Emily. Said to have inspired Charlotte's depiction of Lowood School in *Jane Eyre*, it was immortalised in fiction as a harsh and oppressive institution. While I'm happy to say the school had come a long way since then, I was devastated to be split up from my friends, who were nearly all heading to boarding schools down south.

I went to see the headmaster for an interview. Unlike the cruel Mr Brocklehurst in *Jane Eyre*, he was a kind and encouraging man called Mr Thomas. I thought this would be the perfect opportunity to sabotage the whole plan, so I made a point of saying anything I could to put him off me. When he asked what my interests were, I smiled sweetly and replied, 'Going shopping and being with my friends.'

Something in my grand scheme backfired, because he decided he *loved* my attitude and offered me a scholarship. That meant my parents wouldn't have to pay the full school fees.

Shit.

So, my suitcases were loaded into Dad's lorry, and I was

packed off wearing the most hideous blue school uniform to start afresh. Pre-teens don't really grasp unspoken things like finances or logistics – to me, it just felt like I was being exiled. But this school made financial sense and was half an hour from my brother's, so of course my parents were keen.

Regardless, I made it my mission to get myself out of that school by any means necessary. I started behaving badly, buying cigarettes and pretending to smoke them. I've always hated smoking, but I committed to doing silly, juvenile acts I hoped would get me expelled. I imagined Mr Thomas would regret ever offering me a scholarship. Nothing worked. The naughtier I was, the more he loved my spirit.

Then, halfway through the year, a miracle happened: my brother's school announced it would be accepting girls the following year. Before my parents could say no, I applied. Even at that age, I was headstrong and driven. I can see now what a handful I must have been for them.

I often think about why I was so against going to an all-girls school. Back then, I believed that all girls were bitchy and I got on better with boys. How that preference had embedded itself into my consciousness at such a young age, I can't quite put my finger on, but I'd definitely internalised the idea that other girls weren't to be trusted. French feminist writer and philosopher Simone de Beauvoir believed that jealousy and competition between girls wasn't innate but a product of the patriarchal structures we are raised within. A system that trains us to see each other not as allies but rivals for male attention and approval. In de Beauvoir's *Second Sex*, she explores how we internalise these dynamics early on, often turning our frustrations inwards or against each other rather than at the system that restricts us. Makes sense to me.

I had girl friends at school, and other than the odd comment about my accent or being 'tarty', I'd never experienced mean behaviour. Actually, it was the opposite. And yet, as a child, I still felt like it was cooler to be friends with boys. Somewhere along the way, I'd absorbed the message that being 'girly' was bad or embarrassing. My first boarding school had been very sporty and the teachers used to mock girls from other schools who weren't into games. If it rained, they'd joke that sport would have to be cancelled because the girls didn't want to get their hair wet. We laughed along with them, not realising we were being taught to see girls as weak and vain.

At school and at home, I learned that caring about your hair or makeup – or any aspect of your appearance – was frivolous and petty. Girls who dressed up were seen as trashy or not to be taken seriously. So, it's no surprise that I reacted with horror at being sent to an all-girls school. I'd already begun distancing myself from anything overtly feminine.

After transferring to a boys' school, I became part of a very small minority. That dynamic really nailed down all of the early lessons I'd taken in about male superiority and the importance of how boys viewed me. 'Boys don't like girls who wear makeup' was a big one, but the list was endless. 'Boys don't like girls who are too loud, too opinionated, wear revealing clothes, act slutty.' And, of course, the biggest message of all: that what boys liked *mattered most*. When we constantly tell girls what is or isn't desirable to boys, we teach them that *being* desirable is the priority. We make them see other girls as competition.

Don't want teenage girls to wear blue eyeshadow to school? Fair enough. But banning it on the grounds that 'boys don't like it' isn't just lazy, it's harmful.

During this period of my life, I made a conscious decision to step outside the community of girls and reject anything overtly feminine. I wasn't going to be like *those* girls. By my early teens, I had already internalised the belief that women were inferior – and that if I wanted to be accepted, I needed to shun all things feminine. I had internalised misogyny.

Internalised misogyny happens when women absorb and adopt sexist beliefs about themselves and other women – often without realising it. It's what happens when we grow up in a society that values masculinity over femininity. It shows up in all sorts of ways: belittling other women, judging them for how they dress or live, competing with them, or dismissing feminine traits as weak. It's when we view kindness and empathy as 'soft', or when we think being smart and capable means distancing ourselves from femininity.

It also shows up in how we seek male validation. Dismissing feminine interests, prioritising men's opinions, judging women who expect respect from men. Even success in traditionally female spaces is often seen as less valid. That's internalised misogyny too.

Every time we accept double standards, we strengthen them. If we call a woman bossy or emotional for being direct – but praise a man for the same – we reinforce the idea that men are the standard and women are deviations. When we shame women for being sexual, but excuse it in men, we show what we really value. When we expect women to be polite and accommodating while letting men be brash or rude, we reveal what we truly believe.

When you're raised on media, language and norms that devalue women, it's no surprise so many of us end up believing them. Studies show that gender stereotyping takes root as early as age eight, but the most vulnerable period for internalising misogyny is between eleven and fourteen. That was bang on for me – and because I was now at a boys' school with a wildly skewed gender ratio, I think it embedded even more deeply.

I learned a whole new vocabulary to disparage women. I absorbed double standards like gospel. I judged other girls for their 'moral failings'. Movies, TV shows and books all reinforce the idea that femininity is weak or petty. From Wendy and Tinkerbell in *Peter Pan* to Annette and Kathryn in *Cruel Intentions*, the tropes show up again and again. The mean girl is always catty and calculating – like Regina George in *Mean Girls* or Sharpay Evans in *High School Musical*. Girls learn early on not to trust other girls. The patriarchy rewards us for rejecting femininity. Girls who distance themselves from 'girly' traits are often seen as stronger, smarter or more capable. So that's what many of us do.

8.
Pretty Privilege

While there aren't many ways to talk about this without sounding like a dick, I'm going to give it a try. I'm aware that I have 'pretty privilege', which we can define as an unearned and mostly unacknowledged societal advantage that a person has by fitting into the beauty standards of their culture. I'm blonde-haired and blue-eyed and I've worked as a model, so lots of boxes ticked there. But you don't have to be a supermodel to have pretty privilege, you simply need physical attributes that conform to the beauty standards of the society you live in. Being thin or white or having Caucasian hair gives you advantages in most parts of the world due to white supremacy, for example, so lots of you reading this will be walking through life with 'pretty privilege' whether you realise it or not.

However, when you happen to conform to even narrower standards of beauty, it can feel like you've won the genetic lottery. During my time at the all girls school, we would occasionally partner with boys from outside for certain occasions, such as socials (the boarding school version of a Saturday night disco) and school plays. I got the chance to audition for a musical and was so excited because we'd be rehearsing at the boys' school.

At the time, I was a bit of a misfit and going through my goth moment – dressing in Marilyn Manson T-shirts and big baggy jeans as an act of rebellion. I truly had no concept of my looks. My parents had never told me my appearance was anything of note, and as I wasn't a 'girly' girl, I hadn't spent much time peering into mirrors. It just didn't occur to me.

During the first rehearsal, some sixth form boys snuck into the theatre for a rare glimpse of real-life girls. Shortly after, my best friend came running up to tell me that a lot of the older boys thought I was hot and wanted my number (I had a Nokia 3210). I can still remember this moment so distinctly because I couldn't believe they were talking about *me*. Me? Pretty? Me, the misfit, the goth, the little girl who wasn't 'normal'?

Looking back as an adult, it seems deeply inappropriate that seventeen- and eighteen-year-old boys were effectively telling a thirteen-year-old girl they fancied her. At the time, I didn't understand that I was being objectified, but considering I never even *spoke* to any of those older boys, that's exactly what was happening. Of course, none of that crossed my mind then. I just felt special. The *cool* boys liked me. How lucky was I?

Nothing changed when I looked in the mirror – I didn't suddenly see a swan looking back. I didn't see the prettiness they were talking about. But I did begin to understand that there was attention to be gained in being *perceived* as pretty. The problem was I had no tools with which to manage that attention. If a young girl is considered pretty, she will experience both praise and unwanted attention as she grows up. Compliments can boost confidence, but they also teach her that the way she looks and external validation of that is important. When people are allowed to raise you up; they can also tear you down.

I often see discussions about how important it is not to tell a girl she is pretty because she is so much more than that. While I agree with the sentiment and want Ada to grow up knowing that's far from the most interesting thing about her,

I also know from personal experience how challenging it can be to manage the attention that comes your way.

For me, learning that I was 'pretty' was a watershed moment. I'm sure my parents would be the first to say they're not overly affectionate; they show their love in different ways. But I'd struggled with that and had spent a long time seeking affection and attention elsewhere. Now, suddenly, it felt like I didn't have to. Prettiness meant I didn't have to try to belong.

Another aspect of 'pretty privilege' I was completely unprepared for was the envy, competition and cruelty it could invite, especially from other girls. I still remember a comment a girl in my year made after I became official with my second boyfriend: 'It's not fair. Boys only like you because you're pretty. They don't care about brains or anything else.'

That comment crushed me. It made me feel like I had to prove I was more than my appearance, even though, deep down, I already believed I had nothing more to offer. That one sentence told me I wasn't worthy of love. That if I wasn't pretty, no one would see me.

I've always found the 'bitchy mean girl' trope so reductive. But when society pits women against each other for male approval, it's no surprise that girls with certain features become lightning rods for judgement, jealousy or exclusion. And the worst part is, it doesn't matter whether or not you see yourself as beautiful – other people's projections shape your experience of the world. For years, I saw being pretty as a disadvantage. I didn't think I was beautiful, but I believed men liked me because of how I looked – and only that. When they left me, I assumed it must be because the real me wasn't enough. I'd think, *if beauty is meant to be so valuable, and even that's not enough to make someone stay, then what must that say about who I am underneath?*

When girls were unkind to me, I always took it to heart. I shrank. I didn't realise that their cruelty might have come from insecurity, jealousy, or their own experiences of being overlooked. I hated being judged for my appearance, but, at the same time, I was terrified of losing the one thing I thought gave me value. It's such a trap. As much as I've benefitted from 'pretty privilege' in certain spaces – and I acknowledge that completely – I also hate how much currency beauty holds. I know how it feels to be reduced to your appearance *exclusively*. I also know how painful it can be to feel invisible as a person, as a human with a personality and a mind in a world so obsessed with image. This is especially true in the age of online dating, where so much of our worth is filtered through an algorithm of swipes and superficial judgements. For as long as we place such enormous value on how we look, it feels like there are no winners.

Girls who are seen as beautiful are objectified, judged or resented. Girls who aren't seen as beautiful are dismissed, overlooked or made to feel like they don't matter. Both are taught to doubt themselves. Both are encouraged to see other women as threats rather than sisters. All women suffer in this system.

If my daughter grows up with 'pretty privilege', I want to teach her how to hold it gently, not with guilt, but with respect. I want her to know that beauty can open doors, but it can also cage you. That her value doesn't live in her reflection. That she is never in competition with other girls. That she should honour and uplift other women's beauty rather than measure herself against it. We are not rivals. We are mirrors.

And I want her to know that being admired for how you look isn't the same as being loved for who you are. She should never confuse one for the other. When I look back, I wish I'd known how beautiful I was *both inside and out*. I wish I'd stepped into my power more. I wish I'd spent less time shrinking to make others comfortable, and more time expanding to make myself proud. Because we are all more than our bodies. We are not ornaments. We are whole, wild, worthy beings no matter the shape of our features. Ultimately, no one is pretty if their soul is ugly.

SLUT
slʌt

noun

a highly loaded and derogatory term for a woman who is perceived to have many sexual partners or who expresses her sexuality openly. Historically used to shame women for behaviours that are either celebrated or ignored in men, the word carries deep misogynistic roots, positioning female sexual autonomy as something dirty, shameful and socially unacceptable. It's a linguistic tool used to control women's bodies and choices. Calling someone a slut isn't just about sex; it's about reinforcing the idea that a woman's worth is tied to her purity, and that her power must be kept in check.

Male equivalent: *player, lad or Casanova*
While these terms exist for men, they often carry positive or admiring connotations, as a man with multiple sexual partners is typically congratulated, not condemned. The word slut has no true male equivalent because it is rooted in a gendered double standard.

FRIGID

ˈfrɪdʒ.ɪd
adjective

derogatory term used to describe a woman who is perceived as sexually cold, unresponsive or lacking desire. Historically weaponised to shame women who say no, don't perform sexually 'on demand', or who simply aren't interested in men, it reinforces the idea that female sexuality should be for male pleasure, and if it's not, something must be wrong.

Male equivalent: There isn't a direct male equivalent. A man who isn't interested in sex isn't called frigid – he's often pitied, excused, or assumed to be stressed or tired. Meanwhile, women are pathologised or shamed. At worst, frigid has been used to justify coercion, assault or emotional manipulation. It's a term designed to police women's sexual autonomy and punish them for having boundaries.

Together, the words above illustrate the impossible double bind women are placed in: punished for being too sexual, and punished for not being sexual enough. Like so many gendered slurs, they expose a culture that seeks to regulate and define women by their perceived availability to men, with no space for true sexual autonomy, nuance or neutrality. It's the 'madonna-whore complex' in linguistic form: a woman is either a *slut* or *frigid*, never just free.

9.
School Slut

Before I started at my brother's school – as just one of thirty-seven girls out of 500 pupils – I met lots of my new classmates at a big party during the summer holidays. I already knew lots of the boys from prep school and through my brother, but it was also a chance to get to know the six other girls who would be in my year. It was my first proper party and one of my first experiences getting drunk on alco-pops. I wore heels and a pink dress and was so excited.

I had newfound confidence about how I looked on a superficial level. But prettiness without confidence or self-esteem is a dangerous combination. It can lead you to seek validation in all the wrong places. By the age of fourteen, my self-worth had already become completely sexualised. I believed my value lay entirely in how I looked – and whether boys found me appealing. Don't forget, I'd been playing Spin the Pencil since I was nine, and still naively saw snogging not as a sexual act, but as something funny – like entertainment. It was a game, a laugh, a way of killing time at boarding school. I assumed that's how everyone saw snogging, because it was my normal. So I decided that I would try to snog as many boys as possible that night. I didn't understand the power those kisses would one day hold.

The problem was the boys at my new school weren't privy to that context. For them, snogging wasn't something girls did for fun. It meant something. It carried weight. And because I'd been open about having kissed boys before, I was branded before I'd even had the chance to introduce myself. I became the designated school slut – and I hadn't even gone a millimetre beyond first base.

I entered my new school with a reputation I hadn't earned. People had made up their minds about me before I'd even put on the uniform. I once walked into the school hall at break when I was fourteen and some of the first fifteen rugby team stood up and shouted in unison: 'Slut! Harlot! Whore! Slag!' They were four years older than me. I can still picture their faces as they shouted at me in front of the whole school.

It's hard to explain what that does to a teenage girl. I tried not to react. I kept my head down and walked out quickly, pretending I didn't care. But, inside, I was crumbling. That walk across the hall felt like the longest of my life. The sound of those words – shouted, spat, weaponised – burned into me. I walked away, willing myself not to cry until I got out of the building. When older boys or men shame you, it gives everyone else licence to join in.

If you've ever been on the receiving end of slut-shaming, you'll know how deeply traumatising it is. It's not just name-calling. It's public humiliation. It's being made to feel like your body isn't yours anymore, like it belongs to everyone else. Their judgement. Their gossip. Their fantasies. It was mostly older boys talking about me, rating me, speculating about what I had or hadn't done. And that was the first time I felt genuinely afraid of them. I'd never been scared of boys before. But, now, I felt hunted. I had become easy prey.

Slut-shaming is a tool of control. It tells girls: don't be too loud, don't be too confident, don't be too free with your body, or you'll be punished. And it works. That fear of the boys made me shrink and made me desperate for their approval. If I could just be the 'good girl', maybe they'd like me. Maybe they'd stop. I know now that I carried a shame that didn't belong to me. And as I got older and started to have sexual experiences, that shame followed me. Often, the boys would try to charm me. Sometimes I'd say no, but they'd push, persuade or coax me into things I wasn't ready for. Afterwards, I'd feel used. Cheap. I'd always blame myself. Over time, that chipped away at my confidence. Boys don't grow up with that kind of shame. Their sexuality — and their reputations — aren't at the mercy of girls. But ours are.

Looking back, I feel heartbroken for that younger version of me. Because I wasn't promiscuous. I wasn't provocative. I wasn't even sexual. But even if I had been, even if I had chosen to explore sex, pleasure or desire, I still wouldn't have deserved that treatment. None of us do. Girls should be allowed to make their own choices without being shamed for them. Whether we choose to wait until marriage, have sex with a boyfriend, or have messy one-night stands, we should be free to make those decisions without being branded 'sluts', 'whores' or 'frumps'.

I didn't want to be seen as a slut, I wanted to be considered *girlfriend material*. I was infatuated with the idea of being perceived as the pure Reece Witherspoon character from *Cruel Intentions*, as opposed to Sarah Michelle Geller's 'slutty' character. Even into my twenties, I wanted to be the Charlotte, not the Samantha. The portrayal of women in media was always so polarised — you were either virginal and desirable or sexual and cheap. You might have heard of the 'madonna-whore complex', coined by psychoanalyst Sigmund Freud. He suggested that a mix of cultural influences prompted some men to see women in starkly opposing lights. On one side you had the women who were pure, maternal and sexually naïve, deemed suitable for marriage. On the other, the women who fulfilled male sexual desires, perceived as tainted, fallen and too degraded to be publicly connected to. This led to a situation where men could only marry women who would never sexually fulfil them, and only have fulfilling sex with women they would never marry. For women, it's a lose-lose situation either way.

Boys aren't held to these standards. Their sexuality is celebrated. Ours is policed. One of the problems with this double standard is that it leads to an imbalanced power dynamic where so many girls and women feel that, as soon as they have sex, they give away their power. But they are also at the mercy of men who may dump them. If they are cast aside, they will have to live with the shame of having been used and discarded and building up a 'body count'. For men it's simple – have sex or not have sex, they can follow their pleasure without the risk of reputational damage; see also teen pregnancies. When we consider a high percentage of teenage pregnancies are fathered by men over the age of twenty (with some historic research suggesting up to 70 per cent[5]), the shame is very much on the wrong side. I was just a child trying to understand herself, her body, and her place in the world. And I was punished for it.

Men rarely face such rigid classifications. Promiscuity in boys is praised throughout our society. Religion plays a role, too, with many faiths emphasising female chastity but not holding men to the same standards. Some cultures still severely punish women for sex outside marriage while ignoring it in men. It's worth highlighting that there have only ever been 'fallen women' – never 'fallen men'.

At the root of this repression is a fear of female sexual independence – a sexually, socially and financially confident woman doesn't depend on male validation or control, which threatens traditional power structures. Some men feel insecure when women have multiple partners, so society labels them 'untrustworthy' or 'dirty' to keep them in line.

Pop culture reinforces this double standard. In *American Pie* and other teen films, boys are heroes for having sex; girls are shamed. Female celebrities face intense scrutiny over relationships, while male celebs are admired for their 'conquests'. Taylor Swift gets headlines for dating; male stars don't. Add in internalised misogyny and women join in the shaming, keeping the cycle alive.

Slut-shaming teaches girls to feel guilty about their natural and normal desires. Many of us internalise the shame, leading to insecurity and unhealthy relationships.

People often excuse the double standard by claiming men have higher sex drives. But studies show many couples have equal desire – and men are just as likely to have the lower one. What's fascinating is that men and women report sexual history differently when they believe their responses will be shared.[6] Men exaggerate; women downplay. That fuels the myth that men are always up for it. But if women had grown up free of shame and the pressure to be 'pure', how many more sexual partners might we have had? Or not. We'll never know.

When I was thirteen, I was talking with my best friend about one of the boys I fancied in front of her mum. It felt innocent, just someone to get excited about and giggle over in the same way I did about Zac from Hanson or Aaron Carter (niche taste!). We always talked about who we fancied, so it felt normal – not something I needed to say out of adult earshot. But her mum snapped, 'God, you're like a dog on heat.'

The words cut deep, and I felt so hurt. I didn't know it then, but I was being slut-shamed by an adult. It made me feel ashamed. If a grown-up said it, it must be true. It taught me not to speak freely about my feelings.

It was also so confusing, because at the same time we were reading magazines like *J17*, which were full of articles about crushes and even blow jobs. It's where I first learned that 'real women' shaved their pubic hair – because, apparently, hair was gross. I still remember shaving mine, even though I wasn't sexually active yet. The message had already landed: female pubic hair was disgusting, unhygienic and something to remove.

10.
Deflowered

It's fair to say that interactions with the boys was more or less restricted to lessons. We did have certain official visiting hours when we were allowed to mix, but the boys were very quick to call each other 'slimers' if they so much as uttered a word in our direction. Given the fact that boys at school generally tried to avoid us girls, I was shocked when, on Bonfire Night, some of the cool boys from the year above decided to hang out with us.

It was a cold night, and we all stood around chatting as the bonfire crackled, golden sparks flying into the dark sky. My hands were like ice and one of the boys offered me his coat and hugged me from behind. I could smell his scent and feel his warm breath on me. Eventually he spun me around and kissed me, and as he did, younger kids ran around us with sparklers. Some of his friends laughed, but he told me he didn't care. I had butterflies for the first time in my life. Was this the type of true love they spoke about in the Disney films I'd obsessed over growing up? A boy who wasn't embarrassed to be near me? Who liked me enough to hang out with me in front of his friends? Each time he kissed me it sent shivers down my spine.

For that moment, the world blurred. The fireworks, the sparklers, the crowd – it all faded. All that mattered was that he had *chosen* me. And then, as if the night couldn't get any more surreal, he asked for my number. When I got back to my house, he'd already text me telling me that he really liked me. 'I know you're a player, you probably say that to all the girls,' I replied. 'I don't,' he said. 'I'll prove it. I'll wait for you after church tomorrow.' I couldn't believe it. No guy would wait for a girl after church and risk being forever labelled a slimer in front of the entire school.

But he did. From church, we walked together out in the open, chatting and giggling until lunch. After that, it was officially visiting hours. This meant that girls and boys were allowed to mingle in each other's boarding houses. He came to ours. There were about eight girls in the common room, a couple of boys and him. He put his arm around me as we watched TV. I felt so special. Unfortunately, our housemistress evicted him for breaking the 'six-inch' rule. 'Let's go to my house,' he said. But the same thing happened there – kicked out for holding hands. He then suggested we go somewhere the teachers wouldn't be able to see us. So, we made our way down to the furthest end of the grounds. A place where we could cuddle and snog without teachers kicking us out.

I was totally and completely out of my depth, and, that day, completely unexpectedly, I lost my virginity. I sometimes still feel a sense of shame or discomfort about it even now and I think that's not just because I was so young, but because of my total and complete lack of agency around it. This boy ended up being my first love, and there was no aggression or anything like that. It's just that I didn't have a clue what was happening until it happened. It still feels like it was something that happened *to* me. I often think about how things might have been different had the teachers had a healthier approach to us being together. I understand why they might have been unhappy about two underage kids canoodling, but we were in a safe and public space surrounded by other pupils. The moral of the story? We wouldn't have had sex if we'd been allowed to hold hands.

I do think this story shines an important light on how adults treat teen sex and relationships. Traditional teaching still frames sex as something that happens between two adults solely for reproductive purposes, an archaic perspective that fails to equip young people with the knowledge they need to navigate modern relationships. This rigid and narrow view stands in stark contrast to the messaging we receive from film, television, and even pornography, where sex is often depicted as an act of conquest, primarily for male pleasure, leaving female sexuality as an afterthought.

All the noughties teen films we were watching in the common room exemplified this disconnect. Back to *American Pie* again – the central plot revolves around a group of high-school boys on a mission to lose their virginity before prom, portraying sex as a competitive milestone rather than an experience of mutual discovery. Meanwhile, the female characters are depicted as gatekeepers, with their sexuality tied to emotional attachment. The underlying message is clear: boys should pursue sex at all costs, while girls should only engage in it if they are in love. This dynamic reinforces the idea that sex is something men take, and women give, rather than something both partners experience equally.

The lack of comprehensive sex education leaves us ill-prepared to navigate our own bodies and desires. We worry more about ruining our reputations or what boys will say about our sexual ability. The discourse is always about how good a girl is in bed in terms of how much she satisfies the boy. So many of us enter into sexual relationships with minimal knowledge of our own pleasure, feeling intense pressure to conform to societal expectations rather than understanding what we want. The stakes are disproportionately high for women – socially, emotionally, and sometimes even physically – while men are often encouraged to experiment freely and without consequence.

The result is a culture where women are constantly walking a tightrope: be sexy, but not slutty; be confident, but not intimidating; be experienced, but not promiscuous. Don't be easy, but don't be frigid either. Young women are left to piece together their understanding of sex from a patchwork of conflicting messages, most of which weren't designed with their wellbeing or confidence in mind.

11.
Mind the Gap (in our Sex Education)

Here's what I wish someone had told me about sex:

1. **Consent is Important – and You Can Always Say No**
   Consent isn't just about saying 'yes' once and being locked into something. It's about wanting to say yes, in the moment, and every step of the way. You can change your mind at any time. If someone pressures you, guilt-trips you, or makes you feel like you owe them your body, that's not romance let alone consent. Growing up, consent often meant just resisting long enough, or blaming yourself if you gave in. But let's be clear: the fault never lies with the person who was pressured. Consent should be mutual, enthusiastic, and free from coercion – every single time.

2. **Porn and the Media Do Not Define Real Sex**
   Sex on social media, in movies, and especially in porn is often created through the lens of the male gaze. It's scripted, stylised and unrealistic. It's often performative, not enjoyable. Sex should be about mutual desire, safety and trust. You are not a prop in

someone else's fantasy – you're an equal participant, and your pleasure matters too.

3. **It's Not Your Fault**
If you sleep with someone and they cheat on you, ghost you or brag to their mates – none of that is your fault. Their shitty behaviour is not a reflection of your worth. You are not damaged goods. You are not to blame. If anything, they're the one who should be embarrassed.

4. **Sex Shouldn't Come with Shame**
Shame around sex doesn't prevent girls from being curious, it just teaches them to internalise blame when things go wrong. So many of us entered sexual situations without the tools, language or self-worth to navigate them. In a system that's set up for girls to fail, how can we possibly expect them to thrive?

12.
Schooling in Sexism

The initial introduction of the female of the species into the all-male population of my school was, I'm sure, agonised over. The teaching staff had clearly thought long and hard about how to integrate girls into such an intensely male environment. There were likely all kinds of strategies to make sure our inclusion was seamless and that there were no embarrassing mishaps. Like teenage pregnancies, for example. There had been a huge backlash to the acceptance of girls into the school from former pupils and parents, so it needed to be a success story.

One of the ways they decided to merge girls and boys was by implementing the aforementioned 'six-inch rule'. Cue the boys' crass jokes about 'cutting some off'. It actually referred to the physical distance allowed between male and female students, with the aim of promoting appropriate interactions and upholding the school's standards of conduct.

The main problem with the rule was that it was only ever girls who faced discipline for breaking it. I still remember receiving detention for hugging my brother outside of my boarding house. I was upset, and my brother came to console me, and we got caught breaking the 'six-inch rule'. My brother was sent back to his boarding house immediately and I was reprimanded by my housemistress. 'I don't understand – he's my brother?' I said in disbelief. 'Yes, and do the people in the town know he's your brother? What are they going to think when they see you canoodling with a member of the opposite sex?' I was given detention, but he wasn't. The message was clear: boys could do what they wanted with impunity, but girls had to hold themselves to higher standards.

One evening, one of the boys pulled a moonie at us through the window of our girls' boarding house. If you're unfamiliar with the phrase, it means he dropped his trousers and exposed his bare bottom. It happened a lot at school and was seen as a cheeky joke. One of the girls responded by pulling her top up and flashing him her bra. It wasn't just any bra, either – it was blue with Tweety Pie on it. I imagine one of La Senza's finest. We all exploded into fits of giggles.

What we didn't know was that our housemistress had seen the whole thing unfold from another window. She stormed into the common room and made us all sit down while she shouted at us about how unladylike such behaviour was. There was no mention of the fact that the boy had got his bare bum out. It was, she said, 'different for boys'. There was no question in my mind that this was true. It was acceptable for boys to ping our bra straps through our shirts. It was not acceptable for the girls to react – either through screams or embarrassed laughter. That was seen as attention seeking, and we were told to ignore it and not encourage them. It was acceptable for the boys to snog the girls from the local girls' school at the school socials, but not for us to be caught snogging. If any of us girls succumbed to teenage temptation, we'd be hauled into the deputy head's office and lectured about our morals and our un-ladylike conduct. When I once got caught kissing my boyfriend at the social, the deputy head pointedly told me, 'That behaviour might be normal where *you're* from, but it's not accepted at this school.' Nice little class-based dig there.

One time, a male teacher told me and my friend Kat that while he'd been having lunch in the boys' boarding house, he and the boys had come up with a new sport he was thinking of implementing. What possibly could this new innovation be? It was mud wrestling, he told us with a twinkle in his eye. The premise was that Kat and I would be stripped naked and then slid across the mud. Whoever slid the furthest would win! Why me and Kat? We had the biggest boobs in the school, so I think we have our answer. Instead of disciplining the boys and telling them how completely inappropriate and disrespectful their new sport was, this teacher laughed, encouraged, and then *enjoyed telling us about it*. We were fifteen.

While I walked through the corridors, boys would often run up to me and ask me if I was shaven – in a whisper. The next day, it would be whether or not I liked 'motorboating' (if you don't know what that is, preserve your innocence and don't google it). There was just no escape. Of course, it was all just 'banter'.

There are countless other examples I could share about the daily sexism we experienced during our time at school. Rules set by the boys that went unchallenged by the teachers. Silly things like not allowing girls in the local butcher's shop at break because the 'pies were for boys'. Or deciding one day that girls weren't allowed to enter the communal hall. I once dared to challenge that by bravely stepping into the hall, which was when the first rugby team stood up and heckled me: 'Slut!' 'Whore!' 'Harlot!' Slut shaming is an easy tool to keep women and girls in their place. As a fourteen-year-old girl, that was so affecting. Frankly, I'd be traumatised even if it happened today.

While all this was more than twenty years ago, sexism in school isn't nostalgic – it is still very much alive and kicking today and, according to research, is even on the rise. In a 2024 survey[7] of over 2,000 school support staff, it was revealed that sexual harassment, sexist language and gender stereotyping are major issues in UK schools today. A quarter of respondents working in secondary schools had witnessed sexual harassment over the preceding year. Some examples included:

> Boys touching girls, pushing girls and holding them down to kiss them, playing games called 'rape touch', commenting on girls' bodies.
> Boys commenting on a female student's chest when she sat down opposite them.
> One boy looked up some girls' skirts and made rude hand gestures to them.
> A headmaster text a staff member to say he wanted to see photos of how her operation went. She was having breast enhancement surgery.

In June 2020, campaigner Soma Sara posted on Instagram about her negative experiences of sexism. She then set up a website called Everyone's Invited (now a charity), where young people could anonymously submit testimonials about encounters with sexism in schools and colleges. Tens of thousands of accounts were uploaded, and statistics are bleak: one child is raped in school on every school day.[8] In primary schools alone, three sexual assaults are reported to police daily. Nine out of ten schoolgirls have received unsolicited images or been subjected to sexist name-calling.[9] Put bluntly, there is an epidemic of sexism, and sexual violence, in our schools.

13.
Vulvas for the Win

Looking back, it wasn't long before lots of us were sexually active at school. Surprise, surprise – the 'six-inch rule' didn't work. With that came a lot of unfair bullying and shame targeted entirely at the girls. One girl got with a guy, and he told everyone that she had white spots all over her vagina. She was teased relentlessly. I was horrified – I had tiny white spots on my body too. What if anyone discovered them? Was I abnormal? It turns out that small white spots on the vulva are both very normal and completely harmless. They might be either Fordyce spots – which are actually enlarged oil glands – or vestibular papillomatosis, which is a benign condition where tiny, smooth, skin-coloured or whitish bumps appear on the inner labia or vaginal opening.

Another girl was given the nickname 'Uni' after she hooked up with a guy and he told the whole school that her pubic hair went all the way to her bum – 'like a unibrow'. I panicked – mine did too. I would spend so long on my shaving routine just to make sure no one ever uncovered my horrible secret. Turns out that pubic hair growth around your bum is also completely normal. WHO KNEW? Certainly not me.

When I look back at this level of sexist bullying (all just *banter*, of course), I think of how easily it could have been squashed had we been taught about our female anatomy in school. Both boys and girls were taught about the female parts, but it was in a limited, plain and matter-of-fact way. I was thirty-six before I discovered the correct term for the external part of the female sex organ is actually called a vulva and not a vagina. THIRTY-SIX. We attach so much shame to female genitalia, often telling girls to call it their *minnies* or their *hoo-haas*. The clue is always in the euphemism. Best believe both my children refer to their parts by their actual names, which is slightly awkward when they ask their Gran if she has a vulva (to be fair, she probably doesn't know what they're talking about).

Without proper education, women so often struggle to advocate for their own health or make informed decisions about their bodies. Teaching girls about their reproductive system, menstrual cycle and sexual health equips them with the knowledge to take care of themselves confidently.

Teaching boys about female anatomy and how it functions in non-sexual ways, such as menstruation, childbirth and hormonal health, helps them to see women as whole people, not just as sexual objects. Boys are often only exposed to female anatomy through porn, which is overwhelmingly unethical. The distorted view of women's bodies is truly disturbing, especially knowing that porn is even more accessible to this generation than it was to ours.

Educating both boys and girls about female anatomy is about more than just science – it is about respect, empowerment and equality. When we remove the stigma, we create a world where women feel valued, men become allies, and everyone benefits from a society that prioritises understanding, health and dignity. Us adults have to lead by example, and while it might not feel comfortable at first, it's testicles and vulvas for the win.

DRAMA QUEEN
ˈdrɑː.mə kwiːn
noun

a term used to ridicule someone, usually a woman or girl, for expressing strong emotions or reacting intensely. It reinforces the sexist trope that women are irrational and overly emotional, with a tendency to exaggerate, attention-seek, and it is used to dismiss or belittle genuine feelings around anger, pain or distress.

Male equivalent: While men may be called emotional, they are less frequently shamed for it, and their expressions of anger or intensity are more likely to be seen as justified or powerful. An important exception is that this term is also weaponised against queer or effeminate men who express emotion outside the narrow bounds of stoicism. These men are ridiculed for being 'too feminine', reinforcing the idea that emotion (and women) are weak or inferior. This highlights how both women and queer men are punished for breaking the emotional rules set by a heteronormative, patriarchal culture.

14.
Too Much

I continued to date the boy from fireworks night – he was my first love after all. We hung out whenever we could, and I became borderline obsessed with him. He was good-looking, popular, and he made me feel special in a way that no one ever had before. It was intoxicating and addictive, and for the first time I felt I was experiencing true affection. Even if I got to see him for just a second, I would be giddy. This must be what true love felt like, I thought. I was love-drunk.

Looking back, I realise how unprepared I was for love. No one had ever taught me what a healthy relationship should feel like, or that I didn't have to lose myself to be loved. Every story I'd absorbed from books, films and songs told me love was meant to be all-consuming, dramatic, even painful. So, when I felt obsessed, I mistook it for passion and affection.

The first red flags appeared when we went home for the holidays, and he ignored me for weeks on end. I'd find out that he had other girlfriends, but he'd always seek my forgiveness when term started again. It was only when he started to cheat on me with other girls from school that my world really came crashing down. When he finally broke up with me, it felt like my whole world had ended. I begged him to take me back. This was a cycle that repeated itself again and again for months on end.

And because I'd slept with him, I already felt I'd given something away that couldn't be taken back. There was so much pressure to make it mean something – to make it last. Deep down, I thought it was better to convince him to love me than to be the girl the boys whispered about. I'd given him my virginity because I believed what we had was real, and I didn't want to be left as the girl with a 'body count'. I wanted him to be the only person I ever slept with. That's the power of one-sided shame: girls are taught to guard their virtue, while boys are rewarded for collecting ours. A man's value doesn't diminish with the number of people he sleeps with – only a woman's does. What better way to keep us in line than to make us fear being called a slut?

Between trying to navigate teenage heartbreak, my first sexual relationship, being cheated on, being slut-shamed by the boys, punished by the teachers, while also being sexualised because of my body shape on a daily basis, I was drowning day by day. And being told I wasn't 'normal' either, whether at home or school, as I navigated the class divide programmed me to believe I was not enough. That something was wrong with me. That I wasn't *good*.

One day, my body just gave up and I fainted at school. When I came to, I had my legs on a chair and a very worried housemistress looking over me. Every time I tried to sit up, I vomited. I ended up in hospital for a few weeks. I don't think they ever figured out what was wrong with me. Although in hindsight I'm sure I had some sort of breakdown.

But there was one silver lining: a popular boy from the year above happened to be in the same hospital. I'd wheel myself and my catheter to his ward during visiting hours and we'd chat. With no one else around to call him a slimer, he was kind. Meanwhile, under the covers back at my hospital bed, I'd check texts from friends telling me my boyfriend was snogging other girls at socials. 'Such sluts,' I'd think, focusing on the girls, not him.

When I came out of hospital, I was fifteen, a year into my time at the mixed boarding school, and I was not in a good place. I was no longer with my boyfriend, and the heartbreak combined with the persistent sense that I didn't belong anywhere overwhelmed me. I started to self-harm.

When girls are told they're 'too much' or 'not enough' at such a critical stage of their development, is it any wonder we turn our pain inward? Self-harm among young people is rising. In the year ending March 2022, there were over 25,000 hospital admissions for self-harm among eight- to seventeen-year-olds in the UK,[10] the highest for any age group, making up more than a quarter of total admissions. A quarter of teenagers have self-harmed.[11] That's several in every classroom up and down the country.

For me, it offered a sense of control, or at least it helped me to feel *something*. It was a way to release the pressures I felt I had no one to talk to about. Yet, the more I self-harmed, the more ostracised I'd feel. I was now the freak who was cutting herself. When my school told my parents, they were furious at me. They felt that I was ungrateful. They were sacrificing everything for me to go to school and I couldn't even pay them back with being happy.

School brought in an external therapist. She told me I was the saddest case she'd ever seen and suggested I 'go out and see real problems'. I never saw her again, but her words stuck. Everyone else must be right – I was a total fuck-up.

One day, I was walking along a path near school known as Dog Shit Lane, when a boy ran up to me with a red rose. He told me it was from a boy two years above me. I thought it was a prank. Yet another way to humiliate me. Which boy would want me – the fuck-up, damaged goods and broken? Certainly not a good-looking older guy. I threw the rose in the bin and wiped a big fat tear from my eye. However, it turned out he was serious. Someone in his family had self-harmed, and he wanted to make sure I was okay. We didn't get together right away, but, eventually, he became my boyfriend, my Prince Charming. We dated on and off until my early twenties. He 'saved' me – because in those days I believed every girl was waiting to be saved. That was true love, right?

15.
Silly Girl

Because of everything that had come before, in my later teens I still found it difficult to say no to men – I didn't want to be seen as crazy! – and if I did, I wanted to spare their feelings and didn't dare make a fuss. School had taught me to keep quiet and not encourage attention and pressure with any kind of reaction.

I'm about to share my experiences of sexual assault so please do skip this chapter if you need to.

At the age of sixteen, I was walking through the high street of Carlisle town centre when an old man came up to me and asked if I was a model. Laughably, I was flattered.

'No,' I said, with a shy smile.

'You could be, trust me! I'm a model scout,' he said. 'I've actually got my camera now! I could take some photos of you and send them off to the agency in London. They would love you!'

He suggested we pop round the corner onto a quieter road so he could take some shots. I said okay. As he took photos, he kept asking me to pull my top down a little further. Some shots were far away, some really close up. The closer he got, the more insistent he became that I show more cleavage, so the agency could see it, apparently. I sensed I'd been scammed, but I didn't want to make a fuss. He asked for my email address and told me he'd be in touch. I still shudder at the thought of what happened to those photos, but needless to say, I never heard from him. This is the first time I've ever shared with anyone what happened. Because *obviously* it had been my fault. Silly, gullible girl.

When I was eighteen, I moved to Toulouse by myself and found a cheap hostel I could afford to stay in while I looked for a job. On my first day, I went out in search of an English pub. With almost no experience and limited French, I thought a good old English pub might be my best shot. As I walked around the city trying to find The Frog and Rosbif, a man started to follow me. He asked if I needed help, and I politely told him I didn't. He didn't listen. He kept following me, even to the metro station as I filled out my personal details on a travel card application.

Back at school, I had been learning French with a tutor, called Guillaume – he was actually a professional rugby player who tutored on the side. As he was originally from Toulouse, he'd put me in touch with some friends there so I wouldn't be totally alone. Later that day, the hostel called to say someone was there to see me. I assumed it must have been one of Guillaume's friends, but when I got downstairs, it was the man who'd been following me.

He told me to get on his motorbike, and for whatever insane reason, I did. It was silly, and I didn't want to, but I didn't know how to say no. Nowadays, I would have confidence and the words to have firmly told him to leave me alone the minute he first started harassing me. But let's make one thing clear: it is *never* the 'fault' of women and girls for not understanding how to reject a man or say no in the right way. 'Hold on tight,' he said to me, and I was absolutely terrified at the speed we were travelling. It was my first (and last) time on a motorbike. He sped through the city and, before long, the streetlights disappeared, and we were on a country lane.

'Where are we going?' I asked.

'I need to check my emails at a warehouse,' he replied.

I'm not religious, but I've never prayed harder in my life. How could I have been so stupid?

I must have had an angel on my shoulder because, miraculously, he did just go and check his emails. I sat in the warehouse begging him to take me back, telling him my friend would be worried about me. When I got back, Guillaume's friend had indeed called to check in on me and I arranged to meet him immediately because I was so terrified. That night, when I arrived back at the hostel, the security guard told me that my tutor had tried to get into my room. 'My tutor?' I asked? 'Yes, yes,' and he went on to describe the man on the motorbike. I burst into tears.

My new friend took me to his house, and I stayed there for the rest of my time in Toulouse. One weekend, he was going home to his parents' house in the Gers region for a country music festival and told me I could get a paid job in an outdoor bar there. The only issue? I wouldn't be able to sleep at his house because his parents were Catholic, and even though we weren't a couple, they wouldn't approve of me staying. He said I could stay at a friend's house, and I gratefully accepted. I'd earn enough in those four days to survive until I returned to the UK.

One night while I was sleeping, I felt my foot freezing cold and wet. I froze. I could hear boys giggling at the end of the bed. I still don't know what was touching my feet – their mouths, their genitals? I was so incredibly intimidated. I felt helpless as I lay there pretending to be asleep. I didn't sit up or tell them to fuck off. I was scared at what they might do if they knew I was awake. I never told my friend. I didn't mention it to anyone.

While there is no hierarchy when it comes to sexual intimidation and abuse, and even so-called low-level interactions can have a deep impact on a victim, I did also experience a more serious sexual assault a couple of years later. While at university, I was raped. There, I've said it. It's something I've never spoken about, and yet I've thought about it every single day since – increasingly so since having children. It's one of the very worst moments of my life. I've thought long and hard about whether or not I wanted to include it in this book, because even though a long time has passed, and even though I've stopped blaming myself for what happened, I'm still not very comfortable with people knowing or discussing it.

'Why didn't she come forward at the time?'

'Why did it take her so long to talk about it?'

Then there's the inevitable blame game – what was she wearing? Was she drunk? What's her sexual history? Did she say no *clearly* enough? Was she *asking* for it? Why did she put herself in a stupid position?

And admittedly I had put myself in stupid positions many times before. But then every position is a stupid position if a man is capable of rape.

I'm sure many of you are reading this, remembering your own uncomfortable situations, and perhaps still carrying some shame or embarrassment about your naivety.

Silly girl, they will say.

Maybe some of you are thinking that about me.

But this is victim-blaming pure and simple.

Victim-blaming isn't just about people questioning a woman's behaviour more than the man's, it's also our police and court systems. Around the world the judicial system fails women and girls every single day. Whether it's the judge in Italy who concluded a woman gave false signals to the man who raped her in the women's toilet because she didn't lock the door. Or the woman in Ireland who had her dirty knickers passed around the court. More women than ever are reporting rape to police, yet the percentage of prosecutions has dropped from 25 per cent in 1981 to just 1–2 per cent in recent years.[12] Many survivors say the court experience is worse than the rape. No wonder so many of us keep schtum.

So many women worry that they won't be believed. Public perception of rape is warped by misinformation, particularly around false allegations. Yet only 3 per cent of allegations have been proven to be false.[13] That's not zero, but it's worlds away from the unfounded claims that this is common. This is rape culture – a system that blames women, excuses men, and leaves survivors believing the shame is theirs to carry, like some dirty little secret. In parts of the world, women are still forced to marry their rapist, or face crushing shame for being a victim, because society attaches more importance to a woman's 'purity' than a man's behaviour.

I didn't come forward. Not because I thought the police wouldn't believe me, or that the courts would fail me, but because the man wasn't a stranger in a dark alley. He was a friend. And because of that, the only person I blamed was myself. For years. Even after it happened, I was more worried about him not liking me than I was about my own trauma. I was worried he'd tell other people, and everyone would think I was a slag. So, I didn't tell anyone, and I even tried to stay friends with him. I didn't want him – or anyone else – to judge me.

Even now I find it hard to think about him as a rapist. Even though that's what he was, because I wasn't asking for it. In fact, I was literally unconscious. Even now, I'd worry about ruining his life.

Yes, I was drunk. Yes, I was wearing going-out clothes,

having come from a club. But I was with friends – people I trusted. We don't teach girls that, one day, if they get the chance, their male friends might try to rape them. We imagine rapists to be predators on the street, not names in your iPhone. Yet over 90 per cent of rape and sexual assault victims know their attacker.[14] We need to change how we educate and protect women. Let's never forget, one in four women have been raped or sexually assaulted as an adult.[15]

If you've ever found yourself in a situation where you were assaulted or pressured into doing anything you weren't comfortable with – stop blaming yourself right now.

It doesn't matter what you were wearing.

If you had zero drinks or 1,000 drinks.

If you met someone and went back to theirs.

If you said no, and then didn't fight when he persisted.

No means no. Always. No matter what.

I can't tell you that you should speak up, because I didn't.

I can't even tell you that you will get justice, as too few of us do.

But I know for sure it wasn't your fault, just like it wasn't mine.

I've decided to share this story, inspired by Gisèle Pelicot, because the shame is not any of ours to keep.

Someone did that to me, not the other way around.

And as Madame Pelicot so bravely said: *shame must change sides*.

This chapter isn't just for survivors. It's for everyone who wants to live in a world where we stop shaming women for what was done to them and start holding perpetrators – and the systems that protect them – accountable.

16.
Beauty or Brains

Despite the emotional turmoil I went through at school, I became a solid A-grade student who performed well in tests and exams. It didn't really fit the narrative of what everyone thought about me. I was a bimbo/slut/whore, obviously. One day, a teacher told me that if I wanted to be 'taken seriously' I shouldn't focus so much on my looks. And since I did want to be taken seriously – so much – I listened. I wanted teachers to like me. I wanted to feel valuable. I wanted people to see my worth.

One day I stopped doing all the *silly girly stuff* that I'd adopted once I'd thrown away the emo clothing that had previously been my go to. I stopped straightening my hair with the iron (lol), stopped wearing my blue and pink eyeshadows and Dream Matte Mousse foundation. I stopped wearing silly vest tops and replaced them with huge rugby tops. Suddenly, the constant policing stopped. It felt like I was free. I was still having sex with my boyfriend, but the teachers started being nice to me. Once again, I saw that if you rejected femininity, you would be deemed to be more valuable, and you'd succeed. Any girl who didn't, made her own bed and didn't deserve respect.

By the time I started university, I had very strong opinions about what it meant to be a strong woman. I was intelligent and ambitious and worked hard to be taken seriously. I'd swapped *J17* for *The Economist*. I didn't wear much makeup, I didn't wear revealing clothes, and unlike *other* girls, I didn't need more than a couple of minutes to get ready. I was friends almost exclusively with boys – girls were just too much drama. If my boyfriend had female friends who'd had one-night stands – even on their gap years – I'd question his judgement. 'I don't understand why you want to be friends with a girl like that?' I'd ask. I was incredibly judgemental and misogynistic.

At this point in my life, I'd only slept with two guys, and they had both been long-term boyfriends. I believed this gave me moral superiority and made me *girlfriend material*. I had absorbed so many harmful beliefs about gender roles that I saw stereotypical girl behaviour as frivolous and borderline pathetic. I'd been conditioned to be the perfect Pick-Me.

A Pick-Me means that you reject feminine traits, seek male validation or agree with sexist views. You might say things like 'Wow your ex sounds crazy – girls are such psychos', 'I'm not like other girls', 'I don't need ages to get ready because I don't wear makeup' or 'It's so embarrassing watching female comedians, they're just not funny.'

For years I carried these harmful beliefs into my dating life. I'd love to hear guys telling me their ex-girlfriends were unhinged, as it meant I didn't have to be jealous of them. Clearly, in comparison, I was better than them. I wasn't crazy, I was *so* chilled. *SO* chilled. You could be disrespectful about me and other women and I wouldn't utter a peep because I knew it was *just banter*. I'd take it as the biggest compliment when men told me I was different to other women. Other girls were so lame, but not me!

Perhaps you're reading this and you recognise some of these traits in yourself. Perhaps you've already unpicked a lot of these once-held beliefs. Perhaps, like me, you're embarrassed that you ever felt this way. I just want to reassure you that it isn't because you were, or are, a hateful person or some rampant, woman-hating traitor. It's just that, along the way, you followed the signposts the world laid out for you.

On my journey through my teens, I'd learned that male approval equalled protection and validation. If I could make men like me, I would be safe from shame and bullying. I'd learned that male approval and respect was more important than my own identity, feelings, desires or ambitions. It was certainly more important than my connections to other women.

The problem with rejecting surface femininity and hanging out almost exclusively with men who don't like 'those types of women' is that eventually, one day, the same men will discover you *are* a woman. There aren't 'unicorn women' plucked out from the 'sea of psychos' who are distinct from every other female walking this planet. And no matter how much you try to bend and contort yourself to fit into this horribly narrow and bitter model of easy-going femininity, at some point you will reveal yourself. They will tell stories of how insane *you* were, the wild female things you did, and the rules and restrictions you imposed on them. Like asking them to be faithful, for example, or expecting a reply to messages, a base level of communication for any gender.

I had been dating the boy who had sent me the rose on and off since I was fifteen. After I got back from my six weeks working in France, aged eighteen and just before I started university, we were very much on again. In fact, we were totally inseparable. I believed he was my soulmate, the guy who saw good in me even when I didn't see it in myself. He was also the man who introduced me to the female orgasm. Why had no one taught us about *that* at school? It blew my mind that women could experience pleasure like this, because we were only taught about the male orgasm.

Our one major issue was that his friends didn't want me around. In fact, they didn't want *any* woman ruining their juvenile fun. His housemates were the kind of guys who played games like 'find the poo', where one of them would shit in the nightclub and the others would have to locate the turd. *They actually did this.* They would urinate cross-marks on the backs of girls in clubs they deemed ugly, so they wouldn't be tempted to hook up with them later in the night when their beer goggles kicked in. This misogynistic harassment was, of course, 'just banter'.

When groups of men get together, a pack mentality can form, and their language and behaviour can descend into 'locker-room talk', as Donald Trump famously referred to it when caught on camera bragging about trying to have sex with married women and groping others. At football matches, we often hear misogynist chants, like when Phil Foden's mum was called a slag at the 2025 Manchester derby. When we dismiss sexism as 'acceptable banter' on that scale, it allows people to believe it's acceptable to use such sexual language about women. And to those who say, 'it's part of the game' or 'it's been going on since the beginning of time', I'd ask: how would you feel if it were your daughter being targeted by a herd of men? Not that a man needs a daughter to know that women deserve respect.

For as long as we tolerate this kind of language and behaviour, it desensitises us to more overt forms of sexism and aggression and keeps shifting the boundaries of what's acceptable. When casual sexism is widespread, it contributes to a culture that excuses or trivialises violence against women. We saw in the report into Sarah Everard's murder how the normalisation and acceptance, for example, of Wayne Couzens' vile and deeply abusive language in WhatsApp messages – excused as 'banter' – contributed to his going on to commit atrocious crimes undetected. To break this cycle, we really need men to have the tools and confidence to challenge sexism and harassment among their friendship groups. I certainly hope to give my son those tools, ensuring he can be a good ally. Even if he isn't part of this sort of behaviour displayed by boys in school or men at university, he won't be a silent observer either. And for all the scars I bear from my own school days, in retrospect I can see that lots of these boys were just really damaged by bullying and the misogynistic culture of survival at school.

During that first couple of years of university, I tried so hard to get his friends to like me. I'd turn up to my boyfriend's flat and scrub it from top to bottom, only later to find out his friends would have ejaculated on the bathroom floor before my arrival, knowing I'd be on my hands and knees cleaning it as soon as I arrived. They were so incredibly foul, but I didn't have any other frame of reference.

One day, in my second year of university, they decided I was no longer welcome to spend any time with my boyfriend if they were around. Boy time was boy time. They enforced the rule so strictly that I wasn't even allowed to see my boyfriend on his twenty first birthday. I ran excitedly to his house to wish him a happy birthday and give him his presents, but he wouldn't open the door because 'the boys' were there. I had to leave everything on the doorstep. 'I'll call you tomorrow,' he said apologetically through the glass. The fact that he went along with this tells you everything you need to know. And the fact I went along with it shows you how low my expectations and confidence were by this point.

Prior to this, I'd always prioritised hanging out with my boyfriend and his friends, so unless I wanted to sit at home and quite literally wait for my phone to ring, my only option was to meet some new people. I was nineteen at this point and, quite quickly, I built a new, amazing group of friends – boys and girls from both Manchester and London – who were new and exciting, and they didn't poo in nightclubs or jizz on the bathroom floor. I became particularly close with one of the boys who had been experiencing some health issues. He was very popular, fun, and maybe a little reckless, and we would chat for hours on end about life and music.

Two months after the twenty-first birthday incident, it was the end of term, and everyone was celebrating the end of exams. My boyfriend was heading out with all of his friends, so I went out with mine. At this point, we had been arguing a lot about my friendships with other boys, and we'd often debate whether or not a girl and a boy could just be friends. At the time, I wholeheartedly believed that we could have platonic friendships with men. I needed to believe that deeply, because, otherwise, it invalidated nearly all the friendships I'd ever had.

That night we weren't just celebrating the end of our exams; my friend had also found out he'd finally been given the all-clear for his potentially life-threatening health issues. It was huge. We started the night by filling a paddling pool with spirits and cream soda, and then we drank to our futures. The rest of the night is fuzzy, but it ended with me cheating on my boyfriend.

I would love to omit this part of the story, as I carried a lot of shame and guilt about it for the whole of my twenties. But as I'm speaking about the challenges I faced in relationships, it's only fair that I hold my hands up to my own indiscretions.

We have to acknowledge that mistakes are part of being young. This one moment created such deep self-loathing that it dogged me for so many years afterwards. I allowed men to treat me horrendously throughout my twenties, and part of that is because I felt like I deserved it.

I decided I couldn't possibly tell my boyfriend what had happened. I knew the impact infidelity could have on someone's confidence, and I decided – in some kind of panic – that it would be better to break up with him. He would be heartbroken, but at least I wouldn't leave him with trust issues. I only told him a year later when the dust had settled. I was devastated and came to believe that, quite simply, I didn't deserve love. Because everyone had been right all along – I was just a 'bimbo', a 'slut', a 'whore'. He could do a lot better.

WOMANHOOD

WHORE
hɔːʳ
noun

whore is used to shame and control women, reinforcing the idea that female sexuality is something dangerous, dirty or transactional. Its power lies not in the act it describes, but in its ability to strip women of dignity, complexity and respect. It's a deeply offensive and gendered slur typically aimed at women who are perceived to engage in sex work or exhibit sexual agency. Unlike the neutral term *sex worker*, *whore* is loaded with contempt, shame and moral judgement and is often used to dehumanise and degrade women. It reduces women to objects of sexual use and condemns them for perceived promiscuity, regardless of whether sex was exchanged for money.

Male equivalent: *manwhore* or *gigolo*
There is no direct male equivalent with the same historical weight, venom and social consequences. Terms used for men tend to be playful, even celebrated. The double standard is glaring, as men are rarely, if ever, defined solely by their sexual behaviour in the way this word defines women.

17.
Working Girl

I graduated university with a 2:1 and immediately moved to London for the summer. I had a few ideas about what I'd like to do next, perhaps a master's degree in International Development and Africa Studies at Edinburgh – though I wasn't sure how I'd be able to afford it. I'd managed to get through university with a student loan and a part-time job as a lifeguard, and later as a Student Ambassador. But like so many of us, I had already amassed a lot of debt. I didn't know how I'd afford it again without the option of a student loan, so I decided to stay in London and try to find a job instead. I've never struggled with my work ethic and definitely inherited some hustle from my parents, so I was confident that I'd land on my feet somehow.

I responded to an ad on Gumtree and, before I knew it, I was working my first job in business development for marketing and advertising agencies. I was on a salary of £18k, which meant that, after paying rent, bills and travel costs to live in my house share, I was left with about £40 a month for everything else. During my early days in London, I'd regularly have two jobs – something my friends didn't need to do. Most of them were either supported financially by their families or could live in their family homes and avoid paying astronomical rent. Even though some of them weren't working at all, they still had more disposable income than I did. As an adult, I can see the immense good fortune I had at the time: a solid school education, the opportunity to study at a prestigious uni, and the ability to move – just like that – to the capital city. For so many people, these possibilities are entirely out of reach. But because of the circles I ran in, I couldn't see that. I didn't have the perspective. That feeling of always being on the back foot in high society, pedalling harder and harder to try to keep up, was mentally exhausting. Thirteen years on from my first day at boarding school, I was still desperately trying to sustain a position among this group of people. I'm not providing this context to garner any sort of sympathy, purely to explain my experiences as honestly as I can.

Still, I was a grown-up now and determined to make it in London, so I threw myself into interviews for any job I thought I might be able to get with my limited experience and no family contacts. I once applied to be a hostess at a distinguished gentleman's club. *Sounds glamorous*, I thought! I arrived in my best tweed jacket and Jack Wills separates, only to discover it was an open interview – and all the other girls were wearing bandeau dresses. As we were told more about the role, we were informed that we wouldn't *be allowed to sleep with the men on site* – although it was strongly encouraged to have relationships with them after work to keep them coming back.

'How did the job interview go?' my dad asked.

'I think I got it,' I replied. 'But I also think they want me to be an escort . . .'

Of course, if that interview had happened now, I'd have gotten up and walked out. But back then I was so allergic to making a fuss, I carried on and thanked them for the job offer. I never went back.

The next job I applied for was to be a cocktail maker in a fancy bar on Berkeley Square called Babble.

'Can you make cocktails?' they asked.

'Of course!' I lied.

How hard could it be?

Well, it turns out it's really fucking hard – and I didn't make it past the trial shift.

From the age of twenty-one to twenty-five, I juggled two jobs to keep my head above water financially. My day job ran 9–6 p.m., Monday to Friday, and then I spent Thursday and Friday evenings plus weekends at my side job. It was hard, but it felt worth it to make life in London possible. For the first time, I finally felt like I'd found a place where I belonged.

CRAZY
kreɪ.zi
adjective

a term often used to discredit women by implying emotional instability, irrationality or hysteria. While it can describe anyone acting erratically, when used against women, crazy becomes a tool of control to silence, dismiss or undermine them, particularly in relationships or the workplace. It plays into a long historical tradition of pathologising female behaviour and has been used for centuries to undermine a woman's credibility and agency.

Male equivalent: While men can also be called *crazy*, the term rarely carries the same gendered baggage. A man might be described as *mad, genius, eccentric* or even *volatile* – terms that often imply brilliance or power.

18.
'Crazy Ex-Girlfriend'

As I cycled through different jobs, I had romances along the way. While working in business development, my boss introduced me to his friend. I was twenty-three at the time and he was thirty. He pursued me, made me feel special, and I fell madly in love. I felt so grown up as we paraded through London, going to clubs and on romantic weekends away. We had intense sex, and there were times I'd turn up to his house in just a trench coat. But, of course, that wasn't slutty – because we were *in love*.

One day, I discovered that he'd cheated on me. I *always* knew. I'd had my suspicions, although I didn't have the confidence to follow my gut instinct back then; instead I just felt insecure and anxious and begged him for assurance. He started taking his phone with him everywhere, even to the toilet. One morning, he forgot it as he jumped in the shower, and I took the opportunity to confirm my worst nightmare. He'd cheated on me with a model, and all his friends had been there when it happened. Worse still, they'd been planning a weekend away together.

I'm embarrassed to say that I pretended not to know anything for the whole day. We went to brunch and then to the cinema, and I kept thinking that I needed to walk away – but I just couldn't believe that I'd be better off alone. I literally thought my life would be *worse* without a cheating boyfriend.

Later that afternoon, I confronted him out of the blue, and he cried and told me he'd done it because he felt so insecure – that I was *so* beautiful, it was only a matter of time until I realised that I was too good for him. *Eyeroll.*

A few months later, I took him back. We had a great relationship for another year, and I truly felt I'd helped him work through his feelings of insecurity. He was a great guy who just needed assurance and love, and I could give him that in spades! One day, we were off to the pub with his mates but I needed to go to the loo, so he left me in his apartment, and I was to meet him there. As I was about to leave, I heard his laptop pinging non-stop with messages. Something witchy inside stopped me from walking out the front door and told me to go and check who was sending all these messages.

Surprise, surprise – it was the girl he'd cheated on me with the year before. I read through all his messages assuring her that we weren't together and that I was just this 'crazy chick' (why are we always crazy?) he used to date. I left his house and never returned.

As I ran from that place, my mind was spinning, thinking about every little thing that had happened between us. By the time I got back to my flat, I'd concluded that, really, I probably deserved what had happened to me because of what I'd done that one night at university to my ex. It was karma, and I'd got what was coming to me.

For the rest of my twenties, I dipped in and out of relationships. I saw coupledom as not only a sign of success and status but also protection. When I dated powerful men, people couldn't harm me. No one called me a slut if I was linked to a man, and being in a couple was a shield from my past, from my mistakes, from my shame. I fell hopelessly in love every single time, so sure that, this time round, it was going to be the real deal. But even when things were going well, I'd still think about my school boyfriend – you know, the one who saved me, and who I had betrayed.

It's funny because my glasses were so rose-tinted by this point that I'd never remember the parts where he put his friends' rules before me. I'd only ever think of that terrible night when I'd made such a big mistake. We would often rekindle things, especially when one of our romances fizzled out. I'd always hope that it might be the renewal of our love story, because obviously we were meant to be together. But every time he would hold what I'd done over my head and say he could never trust me again – I'd ruined our chance of making a go of it.

Looking back, I was being strung along, then reeled back in, only to be discarded and rejected time and time again. It was this long, torturous cycle of revenge for the terrible thing I did as a student. Sometime towards the end, in my late twenties, we went away on a spa break together and I can remember feeling so excited. Maybe this time he would forgive me, and we could give it another go, properly, as adults. We were both single and there was really nothing holding us back from making it official again.

On the first night, we got quite drunk and at a certain point he turned to me, grimacing.

'What's wrong?' I asked.

'I feel pretty bad. I don't know why I've made you feel so guilty for cheating on me, because I cheated on you *all the time*.'

I felt like someone had punched me full force in the chest. I honestly wasn't sure I was going to be able to breathe.

'At university?' I whispered.

'Yeah,' he said casually.

'Before I'd cheated on you?'
'Yeah.'

This huge fatberg of guilt I'd been carrying – the guilt that made me blame myself for every horrible thing a man had ever done to me – had been created to soothe his ego. A few years later, I was in a Fitness First class, and we had to pair up with someone in the room. I looked at the girl next to me and we put the palms of our feet together and did sit-ups towards each other.

After we finished the circuits, she turned to me and said, 'Ashley?'

'Yes?' I answered, confused.

'You don't recognise me? It's me.' And then she said her name. I remembered her – she had been one of the only girls accepted by the boys in my ex's uni house share, and I'd been insanely jealous of her at the time.

She told me that she'd slept with my ex while he was my boyfriend. A few times. His housemates had all told her I was a psycho (that 'crazy' thing again!). 'I feel really bad about it now,' she said, as I came in towards her crotch for my sit-up. I never did go back to Fitness First.

Strangely, when the reason I believed I deserved to be treated like shit by men evaporated, the feeling didn't go with it. I had cast myself as the villain for so many years that I had permanently taken on a sense that I was undeserving of love. My self-esteem was so low, and I was so desperate for affection, that I would ignore every single red flag. And guess what? If you believe you only deserve shit treatment – that's exactly what you're going to get.

19.
'She Looks like a Girl from Abercrombie & Fitch'

One of the best second jobs I had was as a model for Abercrombie. I say 'model', but we all know that actually meant shop assistant. Somehow, Abercrombie & Fitch had successfully convinced an entire generation into believing that working in retail made you a supermodel. They hired exclusively 'good-looking' people – predominantly white, the boys ripped, the girls skinny. We were all cast in the image of their wildly successful advertising campaigns, shot in black and white by Bruce Weber. The ultra-cool images featured preppy, blue-blooded Americans (basically like posh kids at English boarding schools) lounging in the Hamptons with horses or sailboats in the background. It was pure aspiration – noughties privilege personified. And even though the pay was basically minimum wage, and the hiring policies were horrendously superficial, working there still felt like some kind of aspirational life goal. It was the ultimate social status, at least in my posh circles.

There's no doubt that getting that job validated me. Suddenly, I was cool. And even if I didn't *feel* pretty, I couldn't deny it – I'd been picked by Abercrombie. It was only after I left my other job to join their graduate scheme that I realised working the changing rooms was not the flex I'd thought it was. As we now know, thanks to exposés of their practices, it was a deeply problematic company with indefensibly exclusionary hiring policies and attitudes baked into its culture. But, at the time, I loved being part of it because of the amazing, creative group of people who worked there.

One of the big reasons so many models, actors, dancers and singers worked for Abercrombie was because of their audition-friendly policy – if you were called for a casting while on shift, you could tell your manager and leave without consequence.

Working among these young stars-in-the-making had a massive impact on me. In the midst of all my childhood confidence issues, I'd always dreamt of being a broadcaster or presenter. When I was sixteen, I'd managed to secure an internship at BBC Radio Cumbria, and at university I was part of the news team at University Radio Nottingham, the year we won Student Radio Station of the Year. As part of that accolade, we got invited to a prestigious radio awards show attended by Jo Whiley, Scott Mills and Chris Moyles, all radio royalty. I was completely starstruck, but as my confidence had ebbed away, so too had my ambitions. No one from my hometown worked in entertainment, and at boarding school being on television or radio was seen as more like wanting to be a pop star or a movie star – not a 'real', achievable job. We were encouraged to aim for graduate schemes or to become lawyers or doctors, so I never really considered it a realistic career path.

Working at Abercrombie introduced me to people who were breaking into the entertainment industry and actually achieving their dreams. For the first time, I started to feel that if they could do it, maybe I could too. I just didn't know how yet.

What I did know was that there were no opportunities to

be entrepreneurial or to make a real difference to the business at Abercrombie. The head office was in Ohio, which was a long way from the shop floor in London. After a few months I accepted a job offer as General Manager at Itsu – a company founded by an incredible entrepreneur. Maybe here, I thought, I could make a real impact. 'Have you got experience in the food and drinks industry?' 'Of course,' I lied. Well, I had been a cocktail maker once upon a time in Berkeley Square . . . Yeah, I know what you're thinking. Still, Itsu was an amazing place to work, and I gained so much life- and career-changing experience. But I also found it incredibly stressful because, if I'm honest, I was totally out of my depth.

By this point I was twenty-five, with little to no background in food, especially not food as sensitive and weather dependent as fresh fish. I was in charge of a team aged nineteen to fifty-plus, many of whom had worked in the industry all their lives. I had strong people skills from my previous roles, but let's just say I wasn't an expert in food or fish. I did everything I could to hit the targets, and I was often working double shifts to cut down on staff hours, sometimes going in at 7 a.m. and not getting home until 10 p.m. I was a ball of anxiety from dawn to dusk.

A year later, I was so unhappy that I decided it was now or never if I was going to try and make it in TV. I had managed to save £2,000, which was an astronomical sum of money to me. It gave me two months to make something happen before I'd have to get back on Gumtree. You have to give credit to the foolishness – and optimism – of youth.

I left Itsu on the Friday and by the Monday had already enrolled on a four-day TV presenting course. On the final day, one of the girls I'd become friendly with told me she'd landed a job as an extra on the reality show *Made in Chelsea*.

'Do you want to come along?' she asked.

20.
Posh Totty

Reality TV was definitely not on my manifestation board (we didn't do those back then – but you know what I mean), but a quick google told me that *Made in Chelsea* was produced by a large production company with other shows that were fronted by TV presenters. Opportunity knocks, or so I thought.

When I arrived on set, I settled into my position as an extra in the background of a scene between Louise and Spencer. When I had the chance, I chatted with some of the crew and asked if they could put me forward for any presenting opportunities. Instead, they asked if I'd ever considered being a cast member on the show.

I was hesitant, but I also knew this could be an incredible opportunity that might finally lead to financial security and the chance to get an agent. They invited me back to film a speed-dating scene so I could see how it all worked. After a few minutes, one of the cast members pointed in my direction and asked, 'Who's she?' Not long after, a producer came over and asked if I wanted to jump in and do the speed date.

At the time, all my friends were obsessed with *Made in Chelsea*, as so many people were (and still are). I was more of a *QI* and *Countdown* kinda girl (I know, how the worm has turned!). But I thought it would be funny to do a cameo, not tell anyone, and wait for them to spot me.

Overall, it's fair to say I struggled in that environment, and it knocked my confidence a lot. I know that reality television has come a long way in its duty of care to its contributors. That said, I'll always be grateful for the platform it gave me and the connections I made.

One of the things that motivated me to say yes to *MIC* initially (and to a career on TV more broadly), was the idea that it would make me very rich. All famous people on TV are rich, right? If I could get a recurring role, maybe I could get out of my overdraft, find happiness, and be the successful, fulfilled and lovable woman I was striving to be. A lack of money had dominated my life since university and, as I've mentioned, featured heavily before that too. Growing up, money worries were an ever-present topic of conversation in my family – three kids at boarding school is a choice, but no joke. Maybe *Made in Chelsea* would change that?

Wishful thinking, sadly. When I signed on to the show properly, ironically I began to struggle more than ever. In the first few weeks of filming, I still did temp work on the side – two jobs were nothing new for me. One day I'd be working in a shop in Marylebone, the next I'd be putting flags on seats at Wembley (who knew that had to be done manually before every game?), and the next I'd be handing out shots in nightclubs. I was prepared to do whatever it took to keep afloat in pursuit of my dreams.

But once my first episodes aired, I started getting recognised. I once did a promo job where I had to hand out flyers for a phone company in Ealing in a branded polo top, and people came up asking for photos with 'Ashley from *Made in Chelsea*'. I had to stop doing those jobs shortly after, and not just because of the recognition, but the production company could contractually call you in for filming whenever they wanted, day or night.

In direct contrast to reality TV making me rich, financially it was unsustainable. Like many similar popular reality shows at the time, *MIC* paid £50 per filming session, and I was lucky if I had one or two a week. You quite literally needed a trust fund to afford rent because having a full-time 9–5 career was a non-starter given the nature of the sporadic filming. So many other reality TV veterans have spoken about this before – it's just the way it was.

Within a couple of months, I had to move out of my house share because I could no longer afford the rent. A friend let me stay at his parents' house outside of London and charged me £400 a month, but even at that amount, I worried about whether or not I'd be able to pay it. The irony wasn't lost on me that I was on a show about really rich people while living in my friend's childhood home, deep in my overdraft, catching lifts to his rugby club in Richmond so I could save on train fare.

On top of the logistical pressure, there's the scrutiny. On a show like *Chelsea,* you are inevitably scrutinised both for your looks and your 'character', and that particular spotlight highlighted all my insecurities about not belonging. It felt like everything I had been trying to hide, all the parts of myself which didn't fit in either at home or at school, were being exposed to the whole world. It was also very intimidating going to film with people who already knew each other so well. Being a newcomer in any situation can be an isolating, nerve-wracking experience, but sometimes there's one person in the mix who welcomes you with open arms and, in this situation, that person was Ollie Locke.

DYKE
daɪk
noun

a slang term for a lesbian woman, historically used as a slur. While some women have reclaimed it with pride, *dyke* is still often weaponised to belittle, intimidate or 'other' lesbians – particularly those who present as masculine or challenge heteronormative ideas of femininity. It implies aggression, undesirability and deviance from traditional gender roles.

Male equivalent: Gay men are also targeted with slurs – *fag, poof, fairy* – that shame them not just for being attracted to other men, but for stepping outside traditional masculinity. Like *dyke*, these words attack both gender expression and sexuality, punishing men for being perceived as weak, feminine or non-dominant. Both terms reflect how society polices behaviour that doesn't conform to patriarchal norms. Whether reclaimed or rejected, these slurs show how rigidly we enforce gendered expectations – and how harshly we punish anyone who refuses to comply.

21.
'I Kissed a Girl (and I Liked It)'

'My handbag is fake,' I whispered sheepishly to Ollie, one of the original members of the *Made in Chelsea* cast, who had come out as bisexual (and would later come out as gay). 'Oh God, darling,' he said, 'don't worry about that, most of ours are too,' he reassured me. Knowing Ollie now, I can say with near certainty his bag was not fake. But he always wanted me to feel comfortable and at ease. He has such a good heart. After a while, we started dating and it was amazing; I'd almost call it a healing experience. We'd go on romantic dates to the aquarium, to Winter Wonderland in Hyde Park, to get coffees, or we'd stay in and watch rom coms. He even took me to New York as a surprise, and we did the *Sex and the City* tour together. It was like dating my best mate (who I fancied the pants off), and after all the bad experiences, it felt nice to be with someone so kind.

One of the things that I found tricky was that *everyone* had an opinion about his sexuality, and they weren't afraid to tell me. Even his friends would come up to me when we were out and say, 'Don't tell Ollie I told you this, but he's gay.' Others would ask, 'Doesn't it bother you that he's been with men?' and the truth was no, it didn't bother me. Why would I care about who someone's ex is – male or female? If at that moment he wanted to be with me, that was enough. I told Ollie that I just wanted him to be happy, whatever that looked like. Whether that was with me, or with another woman . . . or a man.

The truth of the matter is that I've always been interested in women as well as men too. This isn't something that I've ever consciously hidden, but as none of my experiences with women ever reached the relationship stage, I never felt the need to come out. Much like a lot of my identity, I struggle to know where I fit in within the rigid labels of sexuality, especially as I'm now in a heterosexual relationship with the father of my children. Bisexual? Pansexual? Sexually fluid? Who knows? I don't label myself.

I'm sure after everything I've told you about my experiences of desperately seeking male validation, this may come as a surprise, but the exploration of sexuality – whether it be mine or my friends' – is never something that has intimidated me. I know from experience how tricky it can be for someone to figure out who they are in such an aggressively heteronormative environment. Heteronormativity is the overriding assumption that male-female relationships are the default, and it was everywhere. It still is.

I first started to question my own attraction when I was eighteen. It was 2005 and that year the social media site BEBO was launched. It looked nothing like the apps we scroll now, but it let you connect with strangers. As I was navigating these new feelings, I decided to set my preferences to being interested in women, and I would chat to other girls freely without the worry of anyone I knew finding out or questioning me.

So many girls struggle to explore their sexuality because

society has long dictated how women should experience desire, and that's generally through a lens that prioritises male pleasure over our own. This was especially true of same-sex female attraction in the mainstream media of the noughties. From memory, there were no lesbian or bisexual female characters in any kind of film or on any TV shows while I was growing up who didn't at least partially pander to male fantasies. Whether it was *Van Wilder* or *The Girl Next Door*, *Euro Trip* or *Not Another Teen Movie* – all films which were played on repeat in our school common rooms and in bedrooms up and down the country – girl-on-girl was only ever about the boys.

It's probably no surprise, then, that on the rare occasions I kissed girls when I was out in school crowds – whether that was a friend or a stranger in a nightclub – it was considered a performance for male attention rather than an authentic expression of desire. I felt stung when girls laughed it off after kissing me. That often left me feeling a sense of shame, isolation and even guilt that, for me, it had been something more.

The fetishisation of same-sex female relationships made it incredibly difficult for girls like me who were genuinely curious about their own feelings toward other women to explore anything. At school it was always dismissed as 'just a phase' or something girls did to turn the boys on. Those clichés delegitimised the real emotions and desires behind those experiences, so I found it easier to repress my feelings. And anyway, 'The One' is a prince, not a girl, and I was just as obsessed as ever with finding my *happy ever after*.

I do often wonder how many more women would be in same-sex relationships had they had the freedom to express themselves more freely in the 2000s. The world has shifted dramatically, and representation today is so much better. We see more same-sex relationships portrayed more accurately in the media, with many shows featuring complex, fully realised lesbian, gay and bisexual characters, with stories that go beyond clichés. Music has also seen a shift in lesbian visibility, with artists openly embracing their queerness, rejecting the male gaze and still finding mainstream success.

While such progress should be applauded, there's never going to be a quick fix for millennia of patriarchal tradition. At the time of writing, same-sex relationships are legal in approximately 134 countries worldwide – thirty-eight of which have legalised same-sex marriage. However, even in those countries, societal acceptance can vary significantly. There are still sixty-four countries that continue to criminalise homosexuality worldwide, with punishment ranging from imprisonment to the death penalty. Queer representation is increasingly under threat in politics around the world due to the rise of right-wing extremism and many far-right politicians use anti-LGBTQ+ rhetoric to mobilise their base, framing queer rights as a threat to traditional values. In both Europe and the USA, right-wing politicians have led efforts to ban books featuring LGBTQ+ themes from school libraries, limiting access to queer narratives for young readers.

Same sex relationships have always existed around the world, no matter what laws and restrictions are enforced on people. I'd love to see future generations be free to explore their sexuality without the weight of shame or judgement. To all my queer friends and readers, I hope you know that by showing up as yourself you are also helping to change the script. I try to be so conscious of language around my kids, never assuming that they will grow to love girls more than boys or boys more than girls. I don't joke about boyfriends or girlfriends, not just because they're children, but because

I don't want to project heteronormativity onto anyone. My priority for them is to grow up happy and loved, no matter who that's with.

22.
Fame Hungry

Being on a show like *Made in Chelsea* brought some incredible opportunities. As a life experience, it's pretty amazing to say I got to be part of a BAFTA-winning series. I got an agent, and it opened doors I'd been desperate to kick down.

On the flipside, I'd hoped that being visible to producers and showrunners would help me step sideways into other areas of TV, but that wasn't so easy back then. I'd get invited to presenting auditions and while they always went well, and I'd get down to the final two, the jobs would most often go to someone without a reality TV background. As I navigated my mid-to-late twenties, I watched friends both in and outside of the industry move forward in life. Some were getting promotions, others were buying homes or getting married. I, meanwhile, felt increasingly like I was floundering, week by week, month by month, trying to make it in showbusiness.

I stayed determined, even when my parents questioned whether it was time to go back to a 'normal job'. I worked hard to stay relevant and find a way to make money, but it wasn't easy. I had a model agent at the time who represented both me and a friend who had broken through as a TV presenter. He'd often send her invites to events and when she'd ask if I was going, I never knew what to say. I hadn't been invited so when I'd check with him, he'd look at me with pity and say something along the lines of, 'Look, Ashley, I used to manage successful supermodels. 'Look, Ashley, I used to manage successful supermodels. Your friend is credible and going places, and you're just a reality star. I would ask if you could go but I have a reputation to protect. They just wouldn't want you there and that's just the way it is.' My friend would always take me as her plus one, but it always made me feel that I didn't deserve to be there in my own right.

That kind of exclusion – the feeling that I wasn't cool or valid enough to even *stand* in certain rooms – was crushing. 'Am I really that bad?' I thought. And the worst part was that it confirmed everything I'd already feared about myself. The red-rope culture of the industry felt like new evidence that I didn't belong. But as painful as it was, it also lit a fire in me. My sense of injustice has probably carried me through more than anything else in life. I thought: *fuck this*. I am a nice person, I'm kind, sociable, polite, and I can hold a conversation with anyone. And I will work harder than anyone else to prove it.

So, I decided to go to the events anyway, with or without my friend – invite or not. I know, it takes a lot of front, but, fortunately, that's one of my assets. What I learned is that just being *seen* at these events gets your name on the list for the next one. It's a domino effect. One night, there was an event for French Connection, a brand I'd worn and loved since I was young, back when they had those naughty slogan T-shirts. My industry friends had all been invited and were being dressed by the label. I wasn't, obviously (my agent had his reputation to protect), but I decided to go anyway. The day before, I bought an outfit in store on my credit card with every intention of returning it afterwards (I promise I don't do this anymore!). No one would know they hadn't dressed me. Genius!

The only problem was that the brand had actually dressed

someone else – the actress Samantha Barks – in the exact same outfit. I could see the confusion and horror on the faces of the brand's PR and her team when we arrived. The next day, all the press coverage was about *us*, with the headline: *That's Awkward*. (You can still google it.) Sorry, Sam – you looked amazing. And sorry, French Connection, for the headache – great event, by the way!

Either way, I took it as a win. Once articles start being written about you, brands suddenly want you at their events. And, eventually, they even start paying you to show up. Which, let's be honest, I really needed.

23.
Sex Sells

Remember I said I left school with the strong understanding that girls who wanted to be taken seriously should reject overtly feminine dressing and beauty standards? The moment I broke through into the public eye (and, yes, I know it wasn't exactly an A-list trajectory), all that flipped. The pressure and expectations around how I should present myself did a total 180.

When I first appeared on *Made in Chelsea*, I wore little to no makeup, casual clothes (usually Ollie's oversized jumpers), and I'd never really thought about my weight. Suddenly, there was a big focus on how I looked. On one of the reunion episodes, when the cast sat in a studio to discuss the season's drama, the presenter Rick Edwards referred to me as 'Fit Ashley' – and it stuck. And with that came a whole new wave of pressure.

Once I entered the world of showbiz, I was explicitly told that I needed to be seen as hot to succeed. I was encouraged to dial up the sex appeal. I'd always been a 'good girl' who wanted to please authority figures – especially those with more know-how than me. I was ambitious, and seeing successful, sexy women thriving in my industry made me feel like I had to give it a shot. Soon I was booking lingerie campaigns with plenty of skin on show. At first, it felt exciting – having my hair and makeup done, stepping into that world. But looking back with over a decade of experience, I know now that women don't need to 'perform' sexiness to succeed – even if the pressure to look a certain way is still very real, just less explicitly stated today.

The problem was the battle growing and growing inside my head. I felt trapped in a whirlwind of contradictions about what it meant to be a successful woman. Growing up, I was taught that, to be taken seriously, I had to cover up, reject overt femininity, and avoid looking tarty. Intelligence and ambition, I was told, were all that truly mattered. Dressing provocatively or, as the *Daily Mail* would say, '*flaunting my assets*', would undermine my credibility. I had been taught that modesty equated to respectability and that was what success looked like.

But, stepping into the celebrity world, I was met with an entirely different belief system. Suddenly, I was encouraged to wear more makeup, show more skin, lose weight, and embrace a highly curated version of femininity – one that existed not just for myself, but for the approval of an audience. The same society that had warned me about being 'too much' now seemed to suggest I wasn't enough.

Before long, I was angsting over how my body looked in a dress, how much I weighed, and how closely I fit into a whole new list of standards that had been set for me. I developed body dysmorphia, obsessing over imperfections no one else saw, chasing an ever-moving goalpost of what I was 'supposed' to look like. I couldn't win. If I covered up, I was frumpy and uninteresting. If I embraced my femininity, I was a vain, superficial 'bimbo'. The contradictions broke me down, leaving me questioning not just my body, but my very identity. What did I like? How did I *want* to look? Who even was I underneath it all?

24.
'Who've You Got the Girls out for?'

This feels like the right moment to address both the elephants in every room: my massive boobs.

When I was eleven, I was desperate for boobs. Desperate. I thought they were the pinnacle of womanhood and beauty. My mum had quite small ones, so I decided I needed a miracle. I used to cut out pictures of women with big boobs from magazines and keep them in my pencil case. I'd pray to God. I even wrote a letter to Santa one year and put it in the fireplace in the dorm in my school in France. Around the same time, my mum bought me my first two bras – including that infamous 'tarty-warty' black one.

I imagine I aspired to have large breasts because of cultural influences and insecurities. The models in adverts, the women on TV and in films – it all seemed to suggest that large breasts made you more desirable. And at such a young age, I probably associated them with maturity, beauty and positive attention.

Well, manifestation works, my friends, because I asked, and the Lord (or was it Santa?) delivered. By the time I was fourteen, I was a 30GG. But, as the saying goes, be careful what you wish for, because I would soon realise that being a big-boobed girl came with a whole host of issues that I was absolutely not prepared for.

It began when I started going to socials. 'You can't wear that,' my housemistress said, pointing at my floral tank top from New Look. 'Why not?' I asked. 'It's too revealing,' she replied. Reluctantly, I sulked back to my room and changed.

'Can I try it on?' my friend asked.

'Sure, but she won't let you wear it out,' I warned her.

Except she did. I didn't understand. Certain clothes were acceptable for her body, but not for mine?

'You have to leave something to the imagination, Ashley,' I was told by the same teacher. 'Boys don't like girls who show off too much cleavage.'

That was all it took for me to start feeling like my body was wrong. I hated it. My big, slutty boobs. And whenever I voiced any of this, my friends would roll their eyes. They couldn't see how the very thing we'd all been told to want came with so many strings attached – expectations, judgements and contradictions too confusing for any young girl to navigate. 'You love it really,' they'd say. But I really didn't.

Before long, I was trying to get out of sports. I hated running past the boys and hearing all the comments about my boobs bouncing. I managed to fake injuries and avoided all sports lessons for nearly two years. I'd gone from proudly swimming 5k for fun and going to the nationals with my hockey team to actively hiding from PE. I just couldn't bear for my body to be seen and scrutinised and objectified. Instead of giving me confidence, my boobs stole it.

In my twenties, I started to model, and the work offered me a financial lifeline. But because of my stats, specifically my bust size, there were jobs I was told I wasn't appropriate for. At a casting for a major sports brand, I was told my boobs were too big. Girls with big boobs can't be sporty, apparently.

During my modelling days, the feedback was often that I was too curvy. Sometimes it was subtle, but more often it was said directly to my face. Once, in Italy, I was torn apart body part by body part within earshot: 'Her hips are enormous! She needs to lose weight!'

I developed dread around dressing for events – especially if I knew there'd be paparazzi. If I showed my boobs, I was slutty. If I covered up, I looked frumpy. There's such a narrow sliver in between. I'd have panic attacks while getting dressed. 'Ashley James flaunts her generous cleavage', the tabloids would write. Was I flaunting my cleavage? I'd think. Or was I just existing in my body? I hated reading the articles about me, because they always treated me as a piece of meat, or more accurately a pair of boobs.

I didn't even like the woman they were writing about, so how could I expect anyone else to like me? It seemed like all I did was wear revealing clothing to brazenly show off my body, when the truth was I just struggled to find clothes that fit. I was lost. And while I hated the attention on my boobs, I felt like I was reduced to them. As if there wasn't anything else of interest about me.

Getting dressed in nearly every context made me feel so self-conscious and I never knew what to wear. When I finally did decide on an outfit that I felt was 'appropriate', the worst part would be walking to my destination and hearing men honking their horns. 'NICE TITS, LOVE!' It made me feel instantly deflated. I'll never be convinced catcalling is flattering because there is nothing that makes me feel more undermined and vulnerable.

The problem is, when you've got boobs the size of mine,

even when you cover up, you still get sexual attention. Even when there wasn't a centimetre of skin on show, men would talk to my chest instead of my face. And it wasn't just men. 'Who've you got the girls out for?' friends would say when I arrived. I still struggle with getting dressed today, but, luckily, I now have a stylist who helps me navigate it. That's a massive privilege, and it's one of the reasons I always try to share my outfits with my online community.

Today, I hear from so many women with big boobs who've spent their entire adult lives feeling like they have to cover up to avoid unwanted attention. What's confusing is that while large breasts are idealised in the media, living with them can be physically, socially and emotionally draining.

I've always been envious that women with small chests can wear low-cut tops or tight dresses without judgement. When you have a large chest, shirts gape, baggy styles swamp you, and even tank tops show cleavage. There's no happy medium. Too loose and you're invisible. Too tight and you're provocative.

And don't even get me started on shopping for bras. The majority of brands out there don't offer extended cup sizes, and those that do are often incredibly expensive. As a teenager, my friends had cute La Senza bras. I had utility granny bras. (No offence to grannies. Is this internalised misogyny and ageism? I'm still unpicking things every day, as you can see.) As I entered my late twenties, I began to feel angry about the hyper sexualisation of the female body and the shame I'd internalised.

Through my work as a model, I discovered lingerie brands that didn't totally break the bank. I started to share them online. I wanted women to know they didn't have to hide or apologise for their bodies. That their boobs weren't symbols of promiscuity. And that being sexualised isn't our fault; it's a societal issue.

What depressed me was that when I shared pictures of myself in lingerie, the backlash was instant. The slut shaming I expected — I was wearing 'tarty-warty' black bras after all. But there was also vitriol accusing me of using fashion for bigger-busted women to get male attention, and disappointingly, so many of these comments came from women. The men, meanwhile, sent flame emojis and unsolicited dick pics. That kind of male attention had *literally* been the *last thing* I'd ever wanted.

I remember thinking that if I could block men from following me, I would. The comments from men were often disgusting, but when I called them out, women would say, 'If you don't want those messages, you should put it away.' That old chestnut. I was 'asking for it'.

The logic that we are 'asking for it' reinforces the idea that women are responsible for male behaviour, and that if we just buttoned up and covered up, we'd avoid attention and stay safe. That's not keeping us safe, it's expecting us to be submissive. We deserve better. Instead of attaching moral judgement to what women wear or our body types, we should be teaching men not to view us as objects. Let's stop blaming women and start holding men accountable.

Men have the freedom to run around topless. They can wear pretty much anything — short of a mankini or a dress — and avoid any real social commentary. Every summer you'll spot lads with their shirts off, casually walking through the streets, and even when they wear impressively short shorts, no one bats an eyelid. Have you ever thought about how unfair it is that they just get to wear clothing with rarely any judgement about their morals or appropriateness?

If women can manage to control themselves around shirtless men without shouting obscenities or assuming they're 'asking for it', is it really so much to expect the same in return?

For girls, the shame starts early, and it usually begins at home with well-meaning parents. How many times were you told that 'you can't go out dressed like that' as a teenager? This clichéd phrase teaches girls a dangerous message: that it's *their* job to control how men respond to them. That if they wear the 'wrong' outfit, they are to blame for any unwanted attention, harassment or assault they experience. It instils the belief that safety comes from modesty, which we know is a lie. Clothing doesn't protect us from male violence. As the vast majority of sexual assaults are perpetrated by men we know, we're just as likely to be assaulted in our PJs or gym gear as in a mini dress. We're not attracting unwanted attention – *men are giving it to us*. Maybe we should tell boys 'you can't go out' instead, so that we have the freedom to dress how we want?

This same message follows us into adulthood. Phrases like 'mutton dressed as lamb' exist solely to shame women for revealing parts of their body as they age, as if the sight of bare flesh after forty-five is going to blind someone.

I wish I could say things were different now I'm in my late thirties, but the comments I get can still be shocking, especially when I'm on TV. During one of my regular segments on *This Morning,* I wore an epic three-piece purple suit by designer Nadine Merabi. It was love at first sight. I was so chuffed to have found a bra that didn't show, I didn't even consider my cleavage. Ironically, I was discussing the objectification of women, after Hannah Waddingham was told to 'show a little leg' by a photographer on the Olivier Awards red carpet. I came off air to a barrage of notifications. I couldn't believe the drama and discussion that had been stirred up by cleavage!

What's depressing is how little the commentary has changed since I first developed breasts at fourteen. 'ATTENTION SEEKER!', 'WHORE!', 'COVER UP IF YOU WANT ANYONE TO TAKE YOU SERIOUSLY.' It's just so demoralising. The suit wasn't even revealing, but, yes, I do have breasts. Whether I've been fourteen, thirty, or even breastfeeding, I can promise you I have *never* wanted attention for my boobs. They are the last thing I want to be defined by, and it's still an everyday battle to accept them.

What's so interesting is that women with small breasts often wish they had bigger ones. It's another societal paradox: too big, too little. Another example of how rigid the box of femininity is that we're expected to fit into, with no grey area in the middle. Maybe one day I'll get a breast reduction. But I hate that the world sexualises boobs so much that I even have to think about changing my body just to feel safe and respected.

25.
A Moment on the Lips, a Lifetime on Your Sense of Self-Worth

Before I discuss my relationship with my body, food and exercise, I want to acknowledge that I am a white woman in a smaller-framed body. While I've lived with deep insecurities about my body, I've never faced discrimination because of my size. My struggles exist within a society that is overwhelmingly fatphobic.

Fatphobia is rooted in the false belief that being fat is inherently immoral, unhealthy or shameful. It creates a world where people in bigger bodies are judged, mocked, excluded and/or denied proper care because of their size. It's why clothing shops often stop at a size 16. It's why fat characters in films are rarely portrayed as desirable, complex or successful. It's why people in larger bodies are told to 'just lose weight' instead of being offered appropriate healthcare. It's why thinness is sold to women as a moral virtue.

I had to dismantle a lot of my own fatphobia in order to not only accept my body, but to live a life free from diet and restriction. Because I had internalised the belief that thinness wasn't just the secret to beauty and love, it was also the key to success.

Of course, we aren't born believing we need to shrink ourselves to be valuable. Instead, we are literally taught to hate our bodies as we grow up, and the messaging is relentless. And, for me, probably like lots of you, it started when I was a little girl.

I can still recall adults, usually my mum's friends, commenting on my eating habits. 'That's a big portion for a little girl!' they'd exclaim. 'When you get to our age you have to be more careful,' they'd warn. 'It will stick to you here and here.' I have vivid memories of my mum eating cottage cheese straight from the pot instead of eating proper meals in an effort to lose weight. At fifteen, I did the Special K diet because 'everyone was doing it'. Say what you want about diet culture, but that has to be one of the most successful marketing campaigns of all time – convincing an entire generation to give up nutritious meals and eat their brand of cereal twice a day to lose some pounds.

I was a teenager during 'heroin chic' era, when Kate Moss famously said, 'Nothing tastes as good as skinny feels.' I read magazines that circled cellulite on women's bodies and shamed women like Jessica Simpson for looking 'jumbo-sized' when she was about UK size 10. I watched films such as *Bridget Jones*, where her weight was the punchline at nine stone. *Friends* gave us 'Fat Monica' to laugh at. I went to the cinema to watch Gwyneth Paltrow in a fat suit in the film *Shallow Hal* – a whole film premised on how horrifying it would be to fall in love with someone in a larger body.

Everything around me reinforced the idea that thinness was the currency of worth, and anything outside of that was treated as failure or a joke. When you really think about it, it's no surprise that most of us are fatphobic without even realising it. We compliment weight loss without knowing the context.

We ask if we 'look fat' in outfits, even when our friends live in bigger bodies than us. We equate thinness with health, happiness and goodness. We fear gaining any kind of weight – often not because of any real medical risk, but because we know how the world treats people in larger bodies. We see thin as desirable, and fat as a personal failure.

And if things were bad growing up, they didn't get easier in adulthood. I was in my twenties when *TOWIE* coined the phrase 'No carbs before Marbs', and it was entirely normal in my friendship group to discuss our diets, food restrictions and plans to be 'good', starting on Monday. Of course, being 'good' meant barely eating, using exercise as punishment, and obsessively standing on the scales every morning hoping that the number would go down. I judged my days by how little I ate and how well I avoided carbs.

For years, I let meaningless numbers control how I felt about myself, whether it was the number on the scale, the number on my clothing labels or the number of calories I consumed. Getting the lowest number possible was always the goal. I squeezed myself into clothes that didn't fit, just to say I wore a smaller size. I ignored hunger cues, tracked every calorie, and beat myself up when I gave in to them. At my worst, I even ate cotton wool balls soaked in orange juice to suppress my appetite. I shudder to think what damage that did to my body now, but at the time I felt proud at this genius way to stop feeling hungry.

When I got my first job in London, I signed up to Fitness First and, the first time I went to the gym, I ran on the treadmill for as long as I could, obsessively watching the calories tick up so I could 'earn' my night out. Of course, given that I was on 'the cotton-wool diet', I fainted. I woke up in the office being carried by two men and offered fizzy sweets.

And yet, the smaller I got, the more I was praised. 'You look amazing! What's your secret?' I'd hear it from friends, colleagues, and sometimes even strangers. *Oh, you know, just hunger, eating cotton wool, and self-hatred.* I wore their validation like some invisible cloak of honour. If my relationship to my body was bad before I entered this industry, it was far worse inside it. Now I was no longer just battling my own beliefs about myself, I was absorbing everyone else's too.

After *Made in Chelsea*, I signed to a modelling agency and quickly started to see my body as a barrier to my success. No one explicitly told me I was too big, but I saw the castings I didn't get and the jobs I lost as signs that shrinking my body would help things go better for me. This internalised belief was reinforced when I *did* get booked for jobs, and I'd get the photos back to see they'd have photoshopped my body to make me thinner.

At events, I obsessed over dressing 'right' because I knew there'd be paparazzi – and with them, objectification in the tabloids. The comment sections were worse. My boobs added pressure. And I can still remember one comment under an article: 'Someone call the WWF to put her back in the ocean.' That sentence lives rent-free in my head, no matter how many times I try to evict it.

Ironically, when I lost weight, someone else commented that I needed to eat a burger. That's how impossible the standards are: be thin, but not *too* thin. Be small, but not obviously hungry. Look palatable.

During all this, I was still in my overdraft. I felt like a failure, so I told myself if I could just be more perfect (aka thinner), I'd earn more, be more respected, be more wanted.

It wasn't just my career. I saw my single status as a failure too. Men didn't want me – at least not after getting to know me. Each rejection felt like confirmation that I wasn't good enough. And, in my head, 'not good enough' meant 'not thin enough'.

So, I tried harder. I restricted more. And as social media grew, I edited my photos to project that same perfection I craved in real life.

But the more I edited, the more I felt like a fraud. When you get used to looking at a filtered version of yourself, your real reflection can feel confronting. My skin wasn't smooth (I had adult acne at the time), my teeth weren't impossibly white, and my waist wasn't impossibly small. The more I edited my photos, the more I worried about seeing people in real life – be it friends in the industry or strangers I came across – because then they'd realise I didn't look like I did in my photos. My whole life revolved around how I looked, what I ate, and how much I could resist. I was constantly calculating, comparing, shrinking. My body was never neutral – it was always a problem to solve. A project to manage. A source of shame.

Eventually, I realised I couldn't keep living like that. I was tired of being small – in every sense of the word – and I could see that by editing my appearance I was also part of the problem. My own self-hatred was leading me to project an unrealistic version of myself onto other women and girls. I had a choice: keep feeding the cycle, or break free. One day I looked down at my body, saw my cellulite, and thought about my teenage self. Who did she need to see? If I felt like this, surely other women did too. Maybe they might feel better if I posted my body unposed and unfiltered. It felt like a radical move, yet it was so simple. I took a photo, pressed post, and without realising it, sparked my own journey of self-love and acceptance. This moment also marked the beginning of building the amazing online community of women who follow me today. It taught me that, in vulnerability, we can find connection. And it all started with some cellulite.

From that day, I told my modelling agency that I would no longer allow my images to be retouched. They warned me it might cost me work, but that was a risk I was willing to take. I started posting more real pictures of my body: bras that didn't fit, jeans that dug in, softness, cellulite. And something surprising happened: the more I showed up as myself, the more confident I became.

I began curating my online world too. I unfollowed anyone who made me feel inadequate. I stopped consuming content that made me think my body was a problem to solve. I filled my feed with people of all shapes, sizes, races and abilities, which served as a wonderful reminder that beauty is not one size fits all. Slowly, it rewired my brain. I stopped thinking mine had to shrink to be worthy.

I started trying to speak about myself the way I would to my best friend. If your best friend constantly told you that your body was disgusting and pointed out all your flaws, they probably wouldn't stay your BFF for long. Yet that's how our own brains bully our bodies every single day. Now, I stop those bullying thoughts in their tracks and correct myself. It takes time, but every time you shut down negative self-talk and your inner fatphobia, you are rewiring your brain. Here are some examples:

> **Bullying thought**: 'Gross, I've got cellulite – I should wear trousers.'
> *Best friend thought*: '90 per cent of women have cellulite.[16] It's not a flaw, a sign of poor health or something to be ashamed of. It's a totally natural part of many bodies, regardless of size, weight or fitness level. Don't let anyone profit from your insecurities.'

Bullying thought: 'Ugh, I look so fat today.'
Best friend thought: 'Firstly, being bigger is no bad thing – beauty comes in all shapes and sizes. Being smaller didn't make you happier or more confident, and it's normal for your body to look like this. You're probably in your luteal phase.'

Once you start to unpick the fabric of diet culture, it all comes unravelling. One of the most liberating things I taught myself is that clothes are supposed to fit my body – I am not supposed to shrink my body to fit into clothes. I can just size up, and literally no one will know (or care). Also, sizing is completely arbitrary because it changes between brands, seasons and styles. And yet I used to let those tiny numbers ruin my day. Now, I wear what fits – and lo and behold, you actually feel much better in your body when your waistband isn't digging into you. It looks better too.

The same goes for calories. Though the government now lists calorie counts on menus in the name of 'health', we're not learning how to nourish ourselves or make truly healthy choices. A syrupy coffee might have fewer calories than an avocado, but which one is going to fill you up, give you fibre, healthy fats and satiety?

I no longer weigh myself or keep scales in the house – well, other than the kitchen ones and the luggage ones to stop me from overpacking! Now, those scales are important. But it's so weird that we've normalised standing on a machine to let a number dictate how we feel about our bodies. The numbers on a scale tell us nothing about our health, our hormones or our worth. The scale doesn't know how strong you are. (And, yes, muscle weighs more than fat.) It doesn't know how late your period is, or whether you've had a big meal. It's a snapshot of gravity — not a measure of value.

And don't even get me started on BMI! I recently went for a full health check, and despite being-fit, eating well and actually feeling good in myself, I was told I was on the cusp of being 'overweight' according to my BMI.

A few years ago, that would have ruined me and sent me back into disordered eating. Now? I just think — how are we still doing this? The Body Mass Index was invented in the 1830s by a Belgian mathematician — not a doctor — to define the 'average' white man. It wasn't created to assess health, and it certainly wasn't meant for women, children, people of colour or athletes. Yet it's still used in doctor's surgeries, for insurance assessments, and for gym plans up and down the country. It's a system that tells girls so underweight they've stopped having periods that they're 'healthy', while telling professional athletes they're overweight. Why are we still using a flawed, racist, sexist, outdated scale to measure people's health?

One of the biggest shifts for me has been my relationship to exercise. As a child, I would play for hours outside on skipping ropes or pogo sticks (yes, I am that old!). I never viewed it as 'exercise' — like all other kids, I just saw it as play. But somewhere along the way, toxic messaging and 'No Pain, No Gain' slogans crept in, and suddenly movement became a chore; something you had to do as punishment. But after I began changing my relationship with food, I began to move my body for joy again and discovered movement I actually liked — activities like boxing, walking, yoga. And because I wasn't punishing myself, I actually stuck with it.

I got over my fear of carbs and I now eat pasta every day because it's my favourite food and it makes me feel good.

Crucially, it keeps me full so I can focus on all the other important things in life.

I won't lie and say that I always love my body or that I never have wobbles. The conditioning is deep. But I catch it now. I remind myself that my body is not a project to fix. That joy, connection and comfort are more valuable than flat abs and restriction. That I deserve to eat when I'm hungry. And I live a life free from diets, restriction and self-hatred. I wish that for everyone.

In a world now dominated by Ozempic headlines and appetite-suppressant trends – where thinness is once again being sold as wellness, wrapped in medical packaging – I'm more committed than ever to reminding women that we do not need to shrink ourselves. Now that I'm a mum, I am more determined than ever to model a better way because I never want Ada to learn that she needs to shrink herself to be worthy. While I'm sure I can't protect her forever from diet culture, one thing I do know is that she will never hear me speak badly about my body. I don't want her to hear me say I've been 'bad' for eating chocolate, and I don't want her to see me skip meals. I want her to know that food is not a moral test and that her worth will never be tied to her waistline.

I think it's just as important for Alfie too, because I don't want him to grow up believing women are only beautiful if they're small. I don't want him to become another man who polices female bodies with throwaway comments. Instead, I want him to know that beauty comes in so many shapes and sizes – and that a woman's value is never about how little space she takes up. I know I can't protect my children from every toxic message the world will throw their way. But I can show them a different path. At home, we talk about how food makes us feel, and we never refer to it as being 'good' or 'bad'. We don't talk about our bodies like they're problems to be fixed. And I understand that all of that starts with how I treat myself.

Thinness didn't bring me health, love or happiness – but it certainly robbed me of peace and freedom. So, now, I choose something different. I choose to take up space. I choose nourishment. I choose to rest when I need it. To eat when I'm hungry. To say no to shrinking. I can now see that the fairest of them all is not the smallest. It's the one who knows her worth.

Food for thought.

SINGLEHOOD

SPINSTER

ˈspɪn.stə^r

noun

an outdated and derogatory term for an unmarried woman, typically older and presumed to be past the age of desirability or childbearing. The word implies failure, bitterness and loneliness – as if a woman's life is incomplete or pathetic without a husband. It positions marriage not as a choice but as a life goal she has *failed* to achieve.

Male equivalent: There is no direct male equivalent with the same negative connotations. An older unmarried man might be called a *bachelor*, but it's a term that often carries a sense of charm, independence or even desirability. In contrast, *spinster* is cloaked in pity and social failure. This disparity reveals how language polices women's worth by tying it to relationship status, while men are allowed to age freely and remain whole without a partner. *Spinster* doesn't just describe a single woman – it judges her. It frames independence as a flaw and reinforces the idea that a woman's purpose is to be chosen.

26.
Running Out of Time

I always assumed I would get married and have children. That's just what you did when you were a grown-up, so I never questioned any other path. We grow up on a diet of Disney and rom coms selling us love stories where 'happy ever after' begins with meeting the love of your life and ends with driving off into the sunset with a husband. See, historically, women were expected to get married – that's where our value lay. We were traded like cattle from father to husband, with the promise of heirs traded for dowries and social status. While our role in society has evolved, it still automatically celebrates couples and pities singles, especially single women. Gender dynamics may have evolved, but societal expectations have not.

When I was with my long-term boyfriend from school, I had a timeline in my head of how things would go. We'd live together during our year abroad when I was twenty-one, get engaged when we left university at twenty-three, and get married by the time I was twenty-six. What with all the mutual cheating, none of that happened, obviously. But the invisible timeline didn't fade. As the months and then years started to tick by, my panic at being off-schedule set in.

During my late twenties, I went through the worst break up of my life. By this point I'd experienced being cheated on, being the cheat, casual rejection, and let's not forget gaslighting. I'd been ghosted and I'd had my dreams and heart shattered into tiny pieces. But this was different. In retrospect, I can see that we were two people who simply weren't right for each other. A toxic combination. Because of our particular mismatch, we had hurt each other in different ways. No one needs to hear the ins and outs, but it was a dark period of my life and, at the end of it, my confidence was non-existent. I felt totally unlovable and completely worthless. I thought I'd never be able to trust anyone again, and I didn't want to risk another heartbreak like that.

That's when the time pressure really started to hit me. I was meant to be settled and married by now! Instead, I was moving out of the flat I'd rented with my boyfriend after just six months, living on the edge of my overdraft and seeing no real professional progress. Friends were getting engaged, promoted and buying houses. I had been competitive all of my life and had such high expectations for myself, and I didn't understand how I was such a failure. I sat on my suitcase with all my life possessions around me, – anti-bac spray in one hand and a J-cloth in the other – and I fell apart. What the fuck was I doing with my life? I had no plan B. I didn't even know where I was going to live.

Suddenly my phone rang: it was Josie Gibson. I'd met her a few times at various industry parties. "Ere, Ash,' she said, 'I saw you guys broke up, what are you gunna do?' I sobbed into the phone, 'I don't know what to do or where to go.' Four hours later, Josie showed up in a van and packed up me, my dog Snoop, and all our worldly possessions, and drove us back to hers, where we lived for the next six months. I often wonder what might have happened to me without the kindness of Josie. We're all waiting for our white knights, but women rescue us far more often. She scraped my self-esteem off the floor and helped me put myself back together.

Even with Josie as my guardian angel, I would be single for the next six years. Almost immediately after hitting rock bottom, I threw myself back into the dating pool. I really hoped that getting back out there would help me heal. But the more I dated, the more my sense of worth plummeted. Looking back on it now, I can see that I was incredibly vulnerable. I had absolutely no defences and believed such horrendous things about myself that anyone could emotionally take advantage of me.

During the first half of my single era, I believed that if I could make myself aesthetically perfect, then a man would fall in love with me. But the more I tried, the more I got hurt. The irony was that, at the same time, I was regularly featured as both *Esquire* and *GQ*'s hottest woman of the week. There was even an article on *GQ* with a guide on 'How to Date Ashley James'. It felt incredibly conflicting. On the outside I was trying so hard to show that I was a catch, an eligible single woman, and yet on the inside I felt I was broken, irredeemable and repellent.

Every time I was let down by a man – as I always was, because my self-loathing clouded every aspect of my energy – it would provide me with more evidence of how worthless I was. The pattern was always the same: men would pursue and woo me and make endless promises of commitment. They'd tell me that I was beautiful and special, sometimes aggressively, for weeks and even months. I would feel the embers of my confidence trying to catch light. Yet, whenever I'd let my guard down and show myself, they'd disappear or else tell me they weren't looking for anything serious. Each time my hopes would grow, and I'd almost imagine that things could be different. Then it would all come crashing down – taking my confidence with it.

The thing is, I did everything 'right'. I played it all exactly by the book. I was never too keen, I was never 'high maintenance'. I kept all of my inner turmoil inside so no one could ever call me 'crazy' again. I asked endless questions about them; I stoked their egos. I made myself small so they could feel big. I accepted seriously sub-par treatment and behaviour. Yet every Valentine's Day I found myself sitting by a silent phone hoping for the guy I was seeing to ask me on a date. Or even just to text me. By the end of the day, I'd eventually cave and text them something very chilled – usually to no response or a 'you too'. One year, I even saw the guy I'd been dating was out with another girl on 14 February. Of course, then 15 February would come along, and I'd act totally cool and nonchalant about this clear rejection, as I didn't want to be seen as too *intense*.

One man did come along and sweep me off my feet. It wasn't romantic at first, we just started chatting and he made me laugh. He was older than me, which gave me a feeling of safety, and after a while I began to fall for him. It felt like I'd stepped into one of those old-school romances you only see in the movies. And then the press found out.

I still remember lying in my bed when I got an early morning phone call from a number I didn't recognise. 'Hello Ashley, I'm the showbiz editor for the [tabloid newspaper]. I have heard a lovely story that you're dating [insert man].' I didn't know what to say. I'd never had to prepare myself for something like this. Not long after, the relationship was over and, despite never confirming it, I was reduced to being referred to as a 'rumoured squeeze' in any article I featured in. Interesting that a man is never anyone's 'rumoured squeeze'.

It felt like I'd worked so hard to be successful in my own right and now I was just an appendage to a man.

Because I wanted to make it on my own merit, I vowed never to have my name attached to someone else's again, and so I ensured I kept my dating life out of the press. But that desire for privacy – combined with my low self-esteem – meant I let men date me in secret. I didn't expect to be taken out. I let it slide when they didn't introduce me to their friends. If they didn't follow me on social media, I assumed I didn't deserve better. I was scared that, if it failed, I'd be just another man's 'rumoured squeeze'. I'm sure it comes as no surprise that I found men who were more than happy with this set up. Each time, I hoped they would see me as 'girlfriend material', but, each time, I was left heartbroken. What I learned the hard way is that if you don't believe you're worthy of respect, you won't get it. You have to set the boundaries that you expect and deserve.

As the years went by, something started to shift in me. I was so fed up with feeling so fed up. All the effort I'd put into chasing perfection had clearly not been paying off. The more I conformed to beauty standards, the further away I felt from confidence. The more I tried to make men like me, the less success I had. All this time I viewed my single status as a failure and proof that I was unlovable. I knew something needed to change, because the internal debates I was having with myself were exhausting.

Slowly but surely I started to take men out of the equation. I had noticed that every time I started to feel even slightly confident again, it would all unravel around a man. I couldn't keep picking myself up every time the rug was pulled from under me. I'd keep these guys at a distance, let that seed of hope take root, open myself up and then *bam*, it would all implode. I'd find myself chasing, even obsessing over these men as I clung to all the promises they'd made at the beginning. I cringe to admit that I behaved this way.

I can see now that my patterns attracted a specific kind of man. One guy I dated played such mind games with me: hot and cold, in and out for months on end. It was like doing the Hokey Cokey, except I wasn't having much fun. He'd stand me up and ghost my messages. Once, I'd arranged a hotel stay and he left me waiting by myself, watching the clock, 8 p.m. . . . 9 p.m. . . . 10 p.m. Then the excuses would come. 'My friend was in an accident, and I had to go with him to A&E', 'I was at an audition in a basement with no signal'. Every time he'd reel me back in, because deep down I really wanted to believe that maybe he was telling the truth. I wish I could go back and shake myself.

'If you don't like me back, *please* just leave me alone. *Please* put me out of my misery,' I once begged. He held my hand and said, 'Of course I like you,' before telling me tortured stories from his childhood that had apparently affected his ability to open up. I was told I needed to be patient. What I wish I knew then is that it didn't really matter whether his excuses were true. It didn't matter if he liked me or didn't. It also didn't matter if he was emotionally distant because of childhood trauma. What mattered was that he wasn't treating me with the love and respect I deserved. Whether he was unlucky enough that unfortunate events kept happening to him, or just a serial liar, the result was the same. He wasn't able to be a good partner to me. Would I want to settle down with a man who disappeared for days whenever he had a life crisis? I don't think my heart could have coped.

During this period, I sent SO many long messages to men who didn't like me back enough. I chased men who treated me terribly as if they were the loves of my life. Looking back, it's hard to understand why – but I think it's because I felt I'd failed as a woman by not finding my life partner. I felt I was running out of time. I felt unchosen, unwanted, left on the shelf. I also couldn't work out why men liked me so much at the beginning and then became repelled when they got to know me. And why I suddenly became so obsessed with them once the affection they had handed out so casually was taken away.

Looking back, it's easy to see why so many of us blame ourselves if we don't find a partner. From the moment we're born, we're told that, to be complete, we must find someone to complete us. That if we're not 'chosen', we've blundered. And when we fail at that goal, there are labels waiting to shame and embarrass us: 'spinster', 'cat lady', *'crazy* ex'.

Women are celebrated when they attach themselves to a man, and ignored, pitied or patronised when they don't. None of us will ever receive a card to celebrate two years since we walked away from a selfish ex. But Susan will get one for her wedding anniversary to Steve, who slept with a stripper on his stag. No one will gift you a fancy Le Creuset pan for moving into a home all by yourself, but Jane can fully upgrade her entire homeware collection because she got hitched to Jason – a man she's lived with for a decade and who no one wants to sit next to at dinner.

The messaging is clear: it's better to be in a relationship with anyone rather than be single. Better to settle down, not be too picky, not leave it too late. Better to be chosen by someone than to choose yourself. And we haven't got long to fulfil our life's purpose. Tick tock, tick tock . . .

27.
Left on the Shelf

During the six years I was single, I lost track of the comments made to my face to shame me for my single relationship status, further reinforcing my own belief that I was unlovable.

'What's a pretty girl like you single for? What's wrong with ya?' a taxi driver once said to me jokingly. It didn't matter that I knew he thought he'd given me a compliment; it still stung. I laughed politely, counting down the minutes until I'd be dropped off at my work event. 'Don't leave it too long,' he said, 'you don't want to be left on the shelf!'

Left on the shelf. Unpicked and unwanted. This would be a phrase I'd hear a lot over my six years. Sometimes I'd even joke about it myself. Curious after hearing this phrase pop up regularly, I wondered which shelf exactly we were meant to be left on, and I discovered that the phrase actually originated in the nineteenth century. Back then it referred to a woman who had never married and was considered too old for anyone to ask. That was a time when that's all women were: goods and chattels to be owned and sold by men, our value decreasing with our fertility. As we aged, our fathers could demand less cold hard cash in exchange for our hand in marriage. Like spoiled milk, we were considered past our sell-by date if we didn't get hitched in our youth. To this day, this is why men are never 'left on the shelf'.

The fact that we still use this phrase to subliminally encourage women to conform to cultural norms, which prioritise marriage, reminds us how deep the conditioning runs. Plenty of women still believe their prospects of marriage diminish as they age. As if they become less valuable as a potential wife, or have missed their window if they haven't met their husband by a certain age. The closer I got to the big 3-0, the more the comments came. 'Still single?' and 'When are you going to find yourself a nice fella?' were invariably the first questions I'd be asked at weddings – usually while seated on the singles table next to someone's recently divorced and definitely creepy uncle. My own mum once randomly suggested I move back up north because, and I quote, 'men would probably think you're a big deal up there'. 'Do you not want children?' she asked desperately.

The message was always clear: for women, being single in your early thirties is still seen as a sign of failure by society. And the blame? Ours. What *is* wrong with us? Why *has* no one picked us? What *is* it that we do to put men off? Why are we leaving it so long?

For the love of GOD, it is so BEYOND TIME that we stopped placing the blame for singlehood entirely on single women. Perhaps men could start shouldering some of the blame? Just maybe? If he's thirty-five and still playing the field, perhaps someone should ask *him* if he's worried about being 'left on the shelf'.

All I'd ever wanted was the happily ever after. 'It's not for lack of trying!' I'd always want to shout back. 'Maybe you're being too picky,' they'd say. 'You're not a spring chicken anymore!' Well-meaning friends would chip in too. 'Love will find you when you're just not looking.' The irony was never lost on me that most often this advice was given to me by people who had definitely been looking and had met their partners on online dating apps. Others would advise me 'not to put so much pressure on it' in the same breath as asking me if I'd met someone *yet*. MAYBE I WOULDN'T PUT SO MUCH PRESSURE ON MYSELF IF YOU STOPPED ASKING ME ABOUT IT!

While navigating all these comments that made me feel like there was something wrong with me, I also had to survive the hell that is the London dating scene. One date really summed up my rock bottom: a radio presenter arranged dinner at a restaurant he got for free with a VIP card, followed by a concert (also free, as he'd got the tickets free through work). He convinced me to go back to his afterwards: 'just for a drink', he promised. Despite me making it crystal-clear that nothing would happen, he became incredibly rude and angry when I refused to have sex – and then he kicked me out. I felt cheap and worthless – but more than anything, I felt angry at myself for going back to his in the first place. I should have known better. And that's the insidious thing: we're programmed to blame ourselves for being 'naive' or 'gullible', instead of placing the shame where it belongs: on men who lie about their intentions. In the taxi home, I realised I couldn't keep doing this to myself. I felt like I was one more heartbreak away from heart failure.

So, I did what any totally sane person would do: packed my bags and booked a flight halfway across the world to Mexico. All on my own. I needed space away from my life, some space from the sad, desperate, confused woman I had become. I needed to put my own happiness first. After all, how could I expect anyone to love me when I didn't believe I deserved love? Old habits die hard, though, and I definitely hoped I'd meet 'The One' on my travels – but actually something better happened. As I slowly shed the layers of shame and self-loathing, I realised how much all these cultural messages had been weighing on me. I was only thirty, for crying out loud! I wasn't 'on a shelf'! And anyway, since that phrase was coined, women have gained the rights and financial independence to buy the whole supermarket!

I needed to remind myself that finding love was not a race or a competition, and there was no prize for the quickest wedding. In the meantime, I had to learn to be comfortable in my own company. It didn't happen overnight, but as I travelled through Mexico and discovered the joy of deciding what I wanted and where to go next, I started to enjoy my own company. I was slowly beginning to understand the difference between being lonely and being alone. In restaurants, I found myself sitting happily next to couples eating in silence, and I couldn't help but wonder if 'happily ever after' was really as rosy as I'd been sold.

CAT LADY
kæt ˈleɪ.di
noun

a stereotype used to describe an older, single woman who owns (or is assumed to own) multiple cats. It carries connotations of loneliness, eccentricity and social failure – implying that a woman without a partner must be substituting human connection with feline companionship. She is framed as pitiful, odd and undesirable. *Cat Lady* reinforces the idea that a woman's primary value lies in her ability to find and keep a partner – and if she doesn't, she must be lonely, mad or both. The term upholds the cultural myth that a woman without romantic love is somehow incomplete.

Male equivalent: There is no real male equivalent. An older, single man with pets might be described as a 'bachelor', a term that often evokes freedom, sophistication or even desirability. The contrast between a crazy cat lady and an eligible bachelor is telling women are seen as failures for being alone, while men are often celebrated for it.

Single woman stereotypes are so ridiculous when you look at them directly and understand where they come from. And yet so many of us fear them and do everything in our power to avoid these labels. The 'crazy cat lady' is one of the most enduring stereotypes: the lonely, eccentric woman surrounded by a clowder of felines, both tragic and laughable. Just ask J. D. Vance, who famously said that the USA was being run by 'a bunch of childless cat ladies who are miserable at their own lives and the choices they've made'. Is it any wonder that so many of us internalise the fear of dying alone and being eaten by our pets?

Beneath the joke is something darker: a historic discomfort with women who live outside the traditional roles of wife and mother. The 'crazy cat lady' jibe arguably dates back to the Middle Ages and the persecution of witches, when the standard image was a post-menopausal woman living alone, with cats. Black cats especially were seen as demonic helpers, yet in reality they were simply cheaper than dogs, making them the obvious companions for women living on meagre resources. In Salem, a city in Massachusetts, known for its historic witch trials in the seventeenth century, cat ownership was used as evidence of witchcraft. Some even believed witches could transform themselves into cats to attack people. After the trials were later exposed as a grave miscarriage of justice, single women with cats went from being seen as evil witches to just . . . pitied. Suspicion softened into mockery, but the message stayed the same: if you were a woman without a male partner, there must be something wrong with you.

I've always felt a kinship with the women they called witches. According to my Granda (my mum's dad), some of my ancestors were among the Birtley witches. At least, that's what our family has always been told. The story was passed down to my mum, who passed it onto me, an oral tradition linking our bloodline. The details have been lost to the sands of time, but the witches were among a group of fifteen women and one man executed after a mass witch trial in Newcastle in 1650. It was one of the largest mass hangings of witches in English history and yet not much is known about it.

Newcastle at the time was reeling from civil war and plague. The city council hired a 'witch finder' from Scotland, who was paid 20 shillings per accusation – about £100 in today's money, a huge sum. A town crier reportedly walked through the streets urging residents to come forward with accusations, shouting: 'All people that would bring in any complaint against any woman for a witch.'

Thirty people were rounded up and imprisoned for a whole year before half were convicted. There were two prisons at the time: Newgate, for residents of Newcastle, and the dungeons of Newcastle Castle for those from Northumberland – my place of birth.

These women were subjected to all sorts of torturous assessments in an attempt to extract confessions. One method used by Scottish witch finders was 'pricking'. Using a long needle known as a 'witch pricker', they would jab the suspected witch. If she bled, she was deemed innocent. If not, she was found guilty. By the end of the trials, fifteen of those women were publicly hung.

Some of these women likely shared my DNA. We'll never know for certain, but I feel connected to them. Their suffering resonates – as does the pain of all the women who came before us, sacrificed at the altar of patriarchal power. How frightening it must have been for them. How unjust! The older I get, the more fascinated I become with the history of women.

Everything we have today is thanks to battles they fought – and too often we forget how intense those battles were. When we allow lazy stereotypes to box women in, we insult the very real history of what these so-called 'crazy cat ladies' endured.

When women started fighting for our right to vote during the suffrage movement in the late nineteenth and early twentieth centuries, the 'crazy cat lady' label was weaponised against us once more. Anti-suffrage propaganda often used cats in political cartoons to undermine and mock our fight to gain the vote, as well as being used to emasculate men. These cartoons showed husbands stuck at home with cats and crying babies as their wives went out to work. It's a reminder that sexist tropes have always been used to keep women silent and obedient. Single or child-free women are a danger to the status quo, because they threaten the cultural norms that keep the patriarchy functioning. There are few things more radical than a woman who is single and happy.

Throughout history, so many women were mocked – and even murdered – for living outside the rules. For being poor. For being childless. They were women who wouldn't obey. They were women like you and me.

If I had been born in the seventeenth century, I might have been burned at the stake. If I had been born in the nineteenth century, I could have been put in an asylum. If I had been born in the late 1800s, I'd have been imprisoned for fighting for equality.

Society would label me as a troublemaker, or a 'difficult woman'. Women like me have always existed, and we've always been punished for it.

And can I let you in on a secret about the word 'spinster'? The word originally referred to a woman who spun wool for a living. It was one of the few jobs unmarried women could do to earn an income, so it was a term that once signified financially independent women. Over time, marriage became a social expectation for women, so 'spinster' took on a different meaning. It became shorthand for an undesirable and left-behind woman. Just like 'crazy cat lady', it evolved to shame us into compliance. But the truth is, many of those spinsters lived rich, fulfilling, self-sufficient lives.

Naturally, once I discovered the joy of being single . . . I rescued a black cat.

28.
The Difference Between Lonely and Alone

Today, single women still face mockery and annoying comments from people who treat female singlehood like it's a sign of failure. We still judge relationships on how long they last rather than how happy or healthy they are. We assume single people are lonely and couples are fulfilled. But single women today also experience something else: freedom. Freedom hard-won by women who came before us, and that is something we so easily forget when we romanticise the past.

I used to declare that I was a 'hopeless romantic' who just happened to be born in the wrong era. With every new heartbreak, I'd fantasise about living in the 1950s, when all men wanted to get married and, I thought, courted young women with respect. I now know to be careful about viewing history through rose-tinted glasses, because while some marriages in that era may have been full of love and respect, many were not. Marriages back then didn't last a lifetime because people had stronger morals or better communication; it was *until death do us part* because women were trapped: legally, financially, socially. They were literally *unable* to leave.

We forget how recently women gained even the most basic rights. For centuries, marriage was essential for a woman's survival. Women only got equal property rights in 1922 and equal inheritance rights in 1925. In Ireland, a woman couldn't even buy a house without a male co-signer until 1976. Until the mid-1970s, we didn't have full access to higher education or legal protection from workplace discrimination, and women were often sacked for getting pregnant. Up to 1975, it was perfectly legal for employers to advertise jobs with two different salaries – one for men, one for women. Even in 2024, the gender pay gap for all employees still sits at 13.1 per cent in favour of men.[17]

In the not-so-distant past, our nannas – and some of our mums – weren't able to apply for a loan or a credit card without their husband's or father's signature, even if they earned more than both. Basically, if you didn't have a man to vouch for you, you were screwed. So, when your grandmother or mother makes pointed comments about your (lack of) relationship status in your thirties, don't forget how different the world looked in the 1970s. She wasn't just raised to believe that female happiness was found in marriage and motherhood, she was economically and socially coerced into it.

Now let's consider divorce. Today's high separation rates are often held up as a sign of moral decline, and a decree absolute is still demonised in some circles. In the early twentieth century, only two in every thousand marriages ended in divorce. Why? Because it was prohibitively expensive, extremely limited in scope, and *only men* could cite adultery or desertion as grounds. After the First World War, women were finally given the right to divorce on the basis of infidelity, and, by 1937, grounds were expanded to include cruelty, desertion and incurable insanity. Before then, your husband could beat you senseless, cheat on you, abandon you without a forwarding address, have you institutionalised, and you were still forced to remain married to him.

We also need to remember that, until 1991, English law still held that a husband could not be guilty of raping his wife based on the belief she gave him permanent consent when marrying him. And the same goes for domestic abuse: no country had laws protecting women from abusive partners until the mid-1990s. That romantic dream of generations of women achieving the 'until death do us part' bit feels a little less aspirational when we break it down, doesn't it?

'So, tell me, what is the secret to your long marriage?' Answer: LACK OF FREEDOM.

By 1971, 50,000 couples divorced every year, and that number doubled by the 1980s. This has tailed off in recent years, but only because fewer of us are marrying in the first place. There are now just two marriages for every divorce each year. Still, we treat divorce like a moral failure. We applaud couples who've been together for decades without asking if they're happy. We throw parties for wedding anniversaries but never celebrate the bravery it takes to leave a toxic relationship. But let me be clear: divorce is not failure. Divorce means freedom, progress and the right to leave. A right we only have thanks to feminism.

Every woman today owes a debt to those who refused to settle, who demanded more, who walked away. The greatest honour we can give them is to live freely – to choose love if we want to, and to choose ourselves if we don't. Even the women who want traditional marriages owe their freedom to the feminists who made that a choice rather than a sentence. Because that's what love should be: a choice. And we deserve to make that choice without the weight of societal pressure.

I'm not for one moment suggesting we shouldn't dream of a forever love. Of course we can hope to meet someone and grow old together. But we also need to take the shame out of the reality that it might not happen, or that it might not last forever. It's okay to grow apart from a partner you marry or have children with. Choosing happiness is not failure. So many of us grow up believing that personal fulfilment and social acceptance are dependent on finding a life partner, as if everlasting love were the only measure of a life well lived. I believe this stops us from choosing ourselves, because we become so obsessed with finding another half that we forget we are whole on our own. All this messaging feels like patriarchal PR – proof that we're still living under the shadow of a time when women had no choice. But it's time to shake it off, as the great Taylor Swift would say, because times have changed.

Women can now have sex outside of marriage without being banished from their community or forced to wear a scarlet letter. Our children are no longer branded 'illegitimate'. We can buy homes without the signature of a man, we can build stellar, lucrative careers and even out-earn men. And we can say 'fuck all of these standards' and live in a house full of cats and souvenirs from our travels, if we want to – and there is very little anyone can do about it except try to make us a laughing stock.

See, contrary to the fearmongering we're fed about singlehood, research now suggests that unmarried and child-free women are the happiest people in society. Given the sacrifices married mothers make, it's hardly surprising that straight married men live longer and report greater happiness than their single peers. Married women, on the other hand, die earlier and report less happiness than single women.[18] In other words, married men quite literally drain our life force, reducing our life expectancy and our life satisfaction. A 2019 study commissioned by Morgan Stanley[19] found that nearly 45 per cent of women aged twenty-five to forty-five will be child-free and single by 2030 – a figure understandably terrifying for many men who have grown up expecting unpaid female labour. You can see why sexist labels are still needed to convince us we're incomplete without a man. Suddenly, being a 'childless cat lady' doesn't seem so bad.

It's worth remembering that feminism changed men's lives too. For centuries, men had access to free female labour, which allowed them to thrive in the public sphere. A wife was cheaper than hiring a maid, a housekeeper or a nanny – and even better, society had convinced women that this 'work' was their natural calling, while persuading the world that it didn't count as work at all. Men could sleep with other women without consequence, while their wives had no power to challenge them. Men could rape and beat their wives, and the law would look the other way. They owned us. They owned our children. So, when some men today complain that women's gains have come at their expense, maybe they're right – feminism has taken something from them.

In reality, there is *nothing* shameful about being alone. There is nothing tragic about building a life you love, whether or not it includes a romantic partner. It is incredibly admirable when someone – man or woman – creates a rich and joyful life, especially in a world built for couples. Finding single joy doesn't mean pretending you don't want to meet someone. It means enjoying the chapter you're in and knowing that there is no deadline. You don't need to settle, and you are not a failure if you are single. You are not behind. You are not incomplete. And as I learned, it's better to be alone than lonely with the wrong person. Better a 'spinster' or 'crazy cat lady' than a wife to a man who expects you to be his maid, mother, cleaner, cook, therapist and nanny. If only I had learned that sooner.

29.
Tick Tock, it's the Biological Clock

In my attempt to take the time pressures away from dating, I want to make it clear that I'm not ignoring reality. Quite clearly, women are not having children in their eighties, and there is a natural fertility window to consider. For many of my friends who are single, their longing to have children – mixed with concerns about fertility – is at the heart of why they feel such urgency to find a partner within a so-called optimal timeframe.

Take the widely cited statistic that one in three women aged thirty-five to thirty-nine won't get pregnant after a year of trying. That statistic comes from French birth records dated between 1670 and 1830[20] – a time before electricity, antibiotics or fertility treatment. As Catherine Gray points out in *The Unexpected Joy of Being Single*, this figure is wildly outdated. Contemporary research paints a far more hopeful picture: today, more women are getting pregnant in their forties than in their teens.[21] (Granted, this doesn't include IVF figures, but it's still telling.)

I'm not in any way trying to dismiss the very real challenges of fertility. I've held friends' hands as they've navigated – and continue to navigate – the pain of infertility. I've reassured them as they lamented not trying earlier, even though they hadn't met a suitable partner at the time. The devastating truth is that conception can be difficult at any age, and there should be more support in place to help people through that reality. Fertility tests and treatment should be freely available, rather than leaving it down to guesswork, shame and outdated societal pressure.

I ended up meeting my partner at thirty-three and got pregnant at thirty-four and then again at thirty-six – too late in some people's eyes, and a 'geriatric pregnancy' by medical standards. But who was I supposed to be impregnated by before that? Was it the guy who seduced me and then disappeared every time he got a job? Or the one who let me travel an hour from my house to his before pretending he'd fallen asleep? The one who said women couldn't be both mums and career-driven? The serial shaggers, the mind-fuckers, the male chauvinists? Which of this stunning line-up of suitors was I meant to persuade to procreate with me? And if I'd had a baby with any of these unsuitable partners and they left – as many likely would have – guess who would've been blamed for my becoming a single mum? Me. It's always us. It's our fault if we don't pick the right man, but if we only meet the wrong ones within the allotted time frame, the blame lies at our door too.

So often it feels like the pressure is placed entirely on women, but I know a veritable army of them who would love to settle down and become mums, but just can't find emotionally available men. What are they meant to do? To every person who says, 'You don't want to be left on the shelf', might I suggest you spend a week in the modern-day dating pool? Good luck!

What's more, when we speak about fertility, we rarely mention men's declining rates. There's mounting evidence to show that sperm quality decreases significantly with age.[22] Male infertility contributes to approximately half of all cases of infertility and affects 7 per cent of the population.[23] Research has also shown that we're in the midst of a male fertility crisis with reproductive problems in men on the rise – from declining sperm counts[24] and testosterone levels[25] to increasing rates of erectile dysfunction[26] and testicular cancer.[27] And yet fertility is still framed as a woman's issue, a clock ticking towards our supposed feminine expiry date.

What we need is not panic but perspective. We cannot tie ourselves to shitty men just because we feel like we're falling behind. I promise you, those men won't magically transform into the father of your dreams once a baby arrives. In fact, they might just become more selfish, more absent, and even less reliable. And if anyone dares to say you're being 'too picky', ask them this: what should we be picky about, if not the person we choose to share our body, bed, home and future child with?

I'm not pretending the decisions around timing are simple, but I am tired of the fearmongering. Of women being the only ones made to feel like failures if we haven't found someone by thirty. The conversation needs to change. We need to stop assuming everyone's goal is to have a baby, and for those who do, stop pretending it's as simple as just deciding when.

The truth is: we cannot just click our fingers and find a good man.

Perhaps we could start to question why that's so hard, rather than blaming our biology?

30.
Decentring Men

The more I started to unpick societal norms and double standards in my late twenties and early thirties, the more I began to solidly identify as a feminist. Yet the more I used my voice on social media, the more I worried that my opinions and attitudes would stop me from meeting a man. Or rather, that men would be put off because I was *too* much of a feminist.

The ex who was unfaithful to me with that model once messaged me out of the blue to tell me I'd struggle to find love or respect from a man because I posed in lingerie online. Cheers, mate! It's fascinating that a man who lied and cheated still felt entitled to advise me on how to live my life – or to school me on respect. But he wasn't wrong about one thing: there are still plenty of people – men *and* women – who've been conditioned to see certain behaviours as unacceptable in women. For them, sharing images of myself in lingerie, even through a lens of self-love and body confidence, meant I wasn't 'marriage material'.

At the time, I felt a huge disconnect between the woman I had become, the one I showed up as online, and the woman I felt I needed to be to attract a man: polite, compliant, pure. I mean, how many men have 'feminist' at the top of their list for a future wife? Not many. On the flip side, I wasn't about to settle for someone with sexist views, and I didn't want to feel like I had to edit myself to be palatable. And yet that's what dating often made me feel I needed to do.

I think the apprehension so many of us feel about expressing feminist views while dating comes from deeply ingrained gender dynamics. Traditional dating scripts cast women in passive roles – we're expected to be agreeable and non-confrontational – while men are expected to lead and dominate. These tired stereotypes pressure us to downplay our beliefs for fear of being seen as 'too much'. But here's the thing: a man who needs you to pretend to be small will never be able to handle how much space you truly take up. So go in loud. Go in proud. Better to find out early if you're sitting across from a fragile little male chauvinist.

I've had men say to me on dates, 'You're not one of those feminist types, are you?' while laughing. If that ever happens to you: run. It's a massive red flag. We should *all* want equality. But feminism is still painted as incompatible with romance. The hairy-armpit, bra-burning, humourless feminist remains one of society's favourite villains. Feminists, we're told, aren't sexy. They're not fun. They take themselves too seriously. What a convenient narrative for the men who benefit from our silence.

I wish I'd had the confidence back then to say, 'Yeah, obviously. Aren't you?'

It is *not* outlandish to want the same opportunities as a man. It is *not* extreme to believe you deserve equal pay for equal work. It is *not* bonkers to believe in the value of maternity leave. If a man can't see that, he isn't the love of your life. Simple as.

During my Mexican travels, I decided it was time to have a break from actively engaging with men. I needed to take men off the menu entirely, and I needed not to be messaging *anyone*. Taking men out of the equation entirely gave me space to breathe and find joy in other things, and it was that void that allowed me to start unpicking many of the social expectations and pressures I'd been buckling beneath. It also gave me what I needed most: peace. I started noticing just how much energy unworthy men had been taking from me – or, more accurately, how much I had been giving away.

I stopped checking my phone, waiting for someone to text me, or wasting energy wondering why someone hadn't messaged me back (did his battery die? Maybe he got mugged? Perhaps he lost his charger?). I stopped posting thirst traps hoping someone specific would see them. I dressed for myself, not the male gaze. It sounds insignificant, but it had a huge impact on my self-worth. For the first time since I was a young child, I was able to prioritise my own needs, aspirations and well-being.

Despite this freedom, I often felt a hole in the pit of my stomach. Suddenly, I couldn't rely on men for compliments or external validation. I couldn't chase the highs of texting someone, or the rush of them texting me back. Without the usual chaos to distract me, I won't lie – at first, life felt . . . quiet. Maybe even a little flat. I missed the emotional rollercoaster of dating: the hope, the disappointment, the rush. But, for the first time, my self-esteem and mood weren't in someone else's hands. I was no longer co-dependent, but now I had to figure out who I was and what actually made *me* happy. Learning to enjoy my own company was a process. Without a plus one, I began to explore how I liked to spend my time: I loved music. I loved feeling fulfilled in my career. I loved punching boxing bags in dark rooms and other forms of cardio. I loved getting lost in books, binge-watching *Sex and the City*, and going off on adventures. While I was away, I did my PADI Open

Water course, and shortly afterwards, my Advanced certificate. It became this unexpected joy – something completely separate from men, relationships or how I looked.

I realised my life was lacking a group of present and available girlfriends (yes, that was probably *Sex and the City*), so I decided I was going to go out and find them. I began reconnecting with women I'd known and liked but never prioritised because I'd been so busy trying to make men like me. I reached out to girls I'd met through friends or exes. I made friends through hobbies and travels. For the first time in years, I built a support network that didn't rely on romantic relationships.

I used to say I had 'so much love and no one to give it to', but I realised I'd just been looking in the wrong places. Platonic love was everything and more. It was stable, affirming and uncomplicated. I didn't have to wait hours for a reply or wonder if they liked me. They just did.

And because I wasn't wasting my energy on bad dates and broken promises, I had time to pursue things that *actually* filled me up. When I got home, I pivoted my career and poured myself into learning to DJ. It went really well. For the first time in my life, I could get out of my overdraft, pay the bills, and build a life on my own terms. I stopped chasing validation and started chasing purpose.

I finally understood that when you learn to be *actually* happy in your single status, you stop settling for bad relationships. You suddenly have a busy calendar full of friends and newfound hobbies. And because you focus on yourself, everything around you flourishes. As much as I still wanted to meet 'The One', or at least *a* one, the penny finally dropped that waiting around for him to turn up wasn't going to make it happen any sooner. I realised I didn't have control of the timing.

Being single isn't all good or all bad in the same way that every relationship isn't all good or all bad. But when you start to actually enjoy your own company, when you're no longer waiting for someone to complete you, there is such a profound sense of liberation.

After about a year of basking in single joy, I felt ready to reconnect with my desire to form a healthy and loving partnership. Decentring men from my life had been the best thing for my peace, but it was time to find a way to let them back in. But there's one thing in learning how to date healthily, and another in actually applying it to your life. That was the part of the puzzle I hadn't figured out yet, and let's just say . . . there were still more lessons to learn and, unfortunately for me, they would play out in the public arena.

NEEDY

ˈniː.di
adjective

a term often used to criticise women who express emotional vulnerability, seek reassurance or desire closeness in relationships. Calling someone *needy* suggests they are overly dependent, clingy or lacking in self-sufficiency. It shames women for having emotional needs, for asking to be prioritised or for setting boundaries that require effort or care from others.

Male equivalent: While men can be called *needy*, *clingy* or *insecure*, they are far less likely to be pathologised for expressing emotional needs. In fact, men are often encouraged to open up more. When a woman is called *needy*, it's usually shorthand for 'too much' – too emotional, too attached, too demanding. The label punishes women for disrupting the emotional imbalance in heteronormative relationships, where women are expected to nurture others while suppressing their own needs. Calling a woman *needy* keeps her silent and self-sacrificing, lest she be seen as unlovable.

31.
Silent Sisterhood Shifts

If decentring men taught me anything, it's how much of a hole I had in my life where my friendship group was meant to be. If my brain had islands like in Pixar's *Inside Out*, then the path to Friendship Island was very rocky. There's such a pressure to have a group of good girlfriends. The narrative goes that the strongest friendships are the ones that last the longest – that we're supposed to have some sprawling girl gang we've known since school. But I didn't grow up with a lot of close female friendships. Going to a school with so few girls probably didn't help. And by the time I found myself single in adulthood, most of the friends I did have were in relationships or different life stages entirely. I could count on one hand the friends who didn't arrange their plans around their boyfriend's or husband's schedule.

There's no doubt that female friendships can become strained as we move through our twenties and thirties, and it feels like something so many of us experience yet rarely talk about in a constructive way. Society places so much weight on romantic relationships and having babies that when some friends begin to tick off those milestones, others – especially those who are single or child-free – can feel left behind. Often, when they try to express feelings of loneliness or rejection after a friend becomes distant due to a new relationship, those emotions are weaponised or dismissed as bitterness.

When I was single, I often wasn't invited to events that were seen as being for couples. And if I was invited, I was expected to contribute the same amount as everyone else, while being given the children's bed or treated like an afterthought. People would unknowingly pity or patronise me, asking about my love life as if I were someone to be fixed by finding a partner. Friends would set me up with random single men, as though simply being single meant I had no other identity or preferences. I often felt lonely, assuming my friends with children were too busy with family life. I didn't stop to consider that they might not have childcare to join me at the theatre, or that they were simply too exhausted after being up five times in the night. If I'd offered to visit them at home instead, perhaps we both would have felt more seen and connected.

Later, when I became a mum, I found myself on the other side of the fence. I felt lonely and misunderstood by some of my single friends. I'd go online and see them all out together, or even on holiday, and wonder why they hadn't mentioned it. When I asked, they would tell me we were just in different life stages. If I was invited out, they would question why I couldn't just leave my baby for the night or join them on a weekend away. They didn't realise that I longed to say yes, but I just couldn't. I desperately wanted someone to offer to come to spend time with me, to just hang out at home. Motherhood comes with the assumption that your needs vanish, that your happiness is now wholly met by your family. But motherhood can feel isolating too, just as singlehood might.

I have felt deep loneliness in both seasons of life. And what I have come to realise is that both sides carry their own challenges. But instead of bringing us closer together, society often drives a wedge between us. This divide benefits the patriarchy, because when women are busy comparing, resenting or misunderstanding each other, we are not questioning the systems that created these pressures in the first place.

Men do not face the same emotional divisions. Men are not mocked for being child-free or pitied for being single. No one tells them they are in the wrong life stage or suggests they should find 'dad friends' to feel understood. Fathers aren't expected to talk about nothing other than their children, and when they do, they are usually praised. They are not defined by their parenthood in the way women often are. The expectations placed on women are much heavier, and the consequences for not fitting those expectations are far more severe.

If you are feeling the weight of loneliness, my advice is to know that it is okay to find new friends. That might mean joining a new hobby or interest group when you are single, or going to baby classes when you are a new mum. Almost all of my closest friends today are women I met in my thirties, both when I was single and when I became a mum.

I have also learned that friendships can be seasonal. You do not need to fall out with someone just because your lives look different. Sometimes, you find your way back to each other. It's natural to gravitate towards people who are going through similar life experiences, but that doesn't mean the love and respect you feel for your other friends has to disappear. I wish more of my friends had taken the time to get to know my children, but I also know that I didn't offer the same interest or effort to friends who became mums before I did.

We are all just trying to do our best. What matters most is that we keep showing up for one another. We do not need to do that perfectly, but we do need to do it with empathy. I wish we lived in a culture where we talked more openly about these challenges, so we didn't all have to carry them in silence.

32.
Backing the Wrong Pony

When the invitation to go on *Celebrity Big Brother* landed in my inbox, it felt like a sliding-doors moment – one that could either change everything or cost me everything. The producers were developing this particular series to celebrate one hundred years since the Suffragette movement, and they were looking for strong women to enter the house. I was flattered to be considered.

That said, I knew that going back into reality TV carried risks, and that wasn't something I took lightly. I understood the game enough to know it could change my currency within the entertainment ecosystem – for good or for bad. If it went well, it could lead to more opportunities and financial security; if it went south . . . it could be career-ending.

It was also a chance for people to get to know the real me – not just the perceived version of me as 'the girl from *Made in Chelsea*'. I suppose I was still searching for external acceptance, for people to see the real me with proud northern roots. I was scared, but weighing it all up, I decided it was a risk worth taking. Honestly, I was also attracted to the life experience. I was in my 'Ashley does adventures' era. Plus, I was an OG *Big Brother* fan – I was fourteen when it first launched and I used to watch it all the time. And I mean all the time, as in live, 24/7.

When the show fee landed in my bank account, it felt like winning the lottery. Overnight, I was lifted out of the cycle of living pay cheque to pay cheque, free from the constant knot of money anxiety that came with it. We throw around the phrase 'life-changing' too easily, but this really was.

In Britain, we're taught that money is something you don't talk about – that it's improper, even impolite, to name your worth. But if you're not from money – or if you're a single woman – silence won't pay the bills. You have to hustle for yourself. To me, feminism includes financial autonomy: the right to stand on your own two feet, to know that money brings not just survival, but freedom and choice. The trouble is, women are so often encouraged to be grateful for what they're given, while men are raised to expect more. Don't ask, don't get – men know this instinctively. But it's something we need to teach ourselves too, because closed mouths don't get fed.

Not everyone was impressed with my decision to go into the house. My dad had always hated *Big Brother*. Even back when I first told him I was going to be on TV, he said, 'Please don't say it's *Big Brother*.' When I said, 'No, it's *Made in Chelsea*,' Mum asked, 'Wouldn't *Geordie Shore* have been more suitable?' Clearly, she'd never watched the show.

When I told Dad I'd be able to buy my own flat in London, he said all the money in the world wouldn't be worth embarrassing myself on television. I invited my parents to the launch, but they refused to come. I felt incredibly hurt by their disapproval, and it meant that I went into the house hoping the other housemates liked me, that the public liked me . . . and that my parents liked me too. Every single day, I hoped I could make them proud and that I could be normal – just like when I was a little girl.

Launch night came soon enough, and I'll never forget how

much my heart pounded in the moments before Emma Willis called my name and it was my time to step out. This was the moment everyone who had ever loved or hated me would find out I was entering the house. There was definitely an element of imposter syndrome too. Going on a show titled *Celebrity Big Brother* suggests you're a celebrity, and that is never a word I would use to describe myself. I imagined people saying, 'Ashley who?' And I wasn't far wrong.

In fact, people questioned who I had slept with to get a place on the show – because, of course, women can only be successful if they've slept their way to the top. It's an accusation never levelled at men. And isn't it telling, that once again the shame is placed on young women rather than on the powerful men who might actually use sex as currency? For the record: no, I didn't sleep with anyone. And honestly, I don't think I'm that good in bed to hold that much sway.

But I also felt excited and lucky to be chosen as part of a line-up of such powerful women. What comforted me was knowing my girlfriends had turned up to the launch to cheer me on. I didn't get to see them, but I knew they were there, and their presence gave me confidence as I stepped through the door.

I set myself two rules before starting the show. One: under no circumstances was I to fall for any man. Two: I would step away from any conversation or attention on my past love life. I wanted the media to focus on Ashley James – not Ashley James the ex of . . . , or the rumoured flame. It was my time. I had worked so hard to get my foot through the door, and I wasn't going to let anything hold me back.

There was only one problem: I had immediate chemistry with a singer in the house. There was absolutely no denying it. No matter how much I pretended I didn't fancy him, I just did.

Shit.

My friends later told me they'd collectively looked at each other the moment I locked eyes with him and said the same thing. Shit, indeed. Rule one was already looking shaky.

When you're locked in a house with nowhere to escape and very little entertainment, it's hard to avoid both that person and yourself. Before long, what was a mild flirtation grown from a teen-like crush had done its damage. Here was my moment to show I was an independent force to be reckoned with, and yet I was cast as a love interest again – and it was entirely my own doing.

I was annoyed with myself for not being able to ignore said crush, and deep down I felt really exposed. I'd made all these positive changes in my life and grown into a strong, fierce woman in all aspects . . . except for my love life. The episode stirred up all my feelings of self-doubt and reminded me that for all my feminism, I was stuck in old patterns. I'd sabotaged myself.

And guess what? Unsurprisingly, things didn't end well. I'll spare the personal details of how it all came crashing down just days after leaving the house, but it honestly felt like I was in a comedy sketch – except the only thing funny was my love life, and I wasn't laughing. I ugly-cried down Oxford Street, furious that I'd let a man take over my senses yet again.

I still really value the time I spent in the house and the friendships that got me through that experience. But it was a harsh reminder that, despite what they show you in the movies, you cannot change anyone. He is not suddenly going to reinvent himself for you, no matter how amazing you are. You do not need to prove your worth to a man as if once he sees your value he will change his ways and commit.

Backing the wrong horse – or pony, in my case – will always lead to the same outcome, no matter how brilliant you are. It was only once I truly believed I deserved more that I stopped chasing crumbs – and stopped mistaking the crumb dispenser for a feast.

The greatest thing from my experience in the house was when I received a letter from my dad. As a viewer, I'd never understood why people got so emotional when they received letters from home on these shows – they'd only been away a couple of weeks. Had they never been on holiday? But my dad wrote and told me that he and my mum were proud of me, and I still cannot describe what it meant to me. I have the letter framed in my bathroom. He also told me to 'stay away from the wine', and I'm still not entirely sure if he meant the alcohol or Ginuwine. I'll let you be the judge of that.

As I mended my broken (and somewhat humiliated) heart, I realised I had a few things to reckon with when it came to the men I found myself magnetically drawn to. I'd managed to keep things under control when I turned the romantic tap off completely. But the moment I twisted it even a quarter-inch, I was back in hot water.

And I didn't want to keep getting burned.

33.
Learning to Love

After trying to dip my toe back into the dating pond and being snapped at by a school of piranhas, I came to the conclusion that I still couldn't trust myself not to make appalling decisions. I was choosing the same types of men again and again and expecting a different outcome, like a hopeful little moth repeatedly flying into the same flame.

So, I did what any self-aware millennial might do: I turned to books. I read anything and everything I could get my hands on about relationships, attachment styles, childhood wounds and red flags in a quest to find inner peace and a healthy way to date. You name it, I probably read it. I even trained as a life coach! It felt like I was studying for a PhD in relationship psychology. These books helped me see how my past had shaped me and how I'd been hardwired to seek out the wrong kind of love. I've listed as many of them as possible in the back pages of this book, in the hope they might help someone else who's been stuck in the same painful patterns.

One of the most transformational books I read was *Attached,* by Amir Levine and Rachel S. F. Heller. It introduced me to attachment theory, which is now widely accepted in psychology. In a nutshell, attachment theory explores how our early experiences with caregivers (usually our parents) shape how we connect with others in adulthood.

There are three main attachment styles: secure, anxious and avoidant.

People with a secure attachment style are comfortable with intimacy and tend to foster stable relationships. Anxiously attached people, like me, crave closeness but constantly fear abandonment, often becoming overly sensitive or seeking reassurance. Those with avoidant attachment prefer independence and often struggle with intimacy, creating emotional distance to feel in control. Learning about the anxious-avoidant trap was a lightbulb moment for me. This dynamic perfectly explained the patterns I kept repeating: being constantly drawn to avoidant men – emotionally unavailable, hot and cold, withholding. And, painfully, they were drawn to me too, with my neediness and endless craving for validation. We mirrored each other's insecurities. I chased; they retreated. I craved closeness; they pulled away. And the more I pursued, the more they confirmed my deepest fear: that I wasn't enough.

That's the thing with attachment wounds – they feel familiar. For anxiously attached people, an avoidant partner can feel like home, because that was often what love looked like in childhood. Unpredictable. Inconsistent. Something you had to earn. Like the little girl who didn't feel normal at home or school, always trying to prove her worth and value to both worlds. And so I spent years, unknowingly, trying to prove I was lovable. Trying to convince people who couldn't or wouldn't choose me that I was worth choosing. And, of course, when someone finally did give me attention, I confused that for love. I confused intensity for intimacy.

Another book that helped me untangle things was *The Five Love Languages*, by Dr Gary Chapman. He's identified five ways we all express and receive love: words of affirmation, quality time, receiving gifts, acts of service and physical touch. The theory suggests that we need to understand each other's language to be able to have a loving relationship. What resonated most wasn't just how this applied to romantic relationships, but how it helped me understand my own relationship with my parents, especially my mum.

Like so many women, I've had a complicated relationship with the woman who made me. She's a hardened Northern grafter, not naturally affectionate, and always busy providing. As a kid, I didn't understand that her love language was Acts of Service. She wasn't going to wrap me in hugs and tell me I was wonderful. But she'd be up at 6 a.m. making packed lunches, serving breakfasts at our B&B, running her salon, ironing my dad's shirts, and hunting through her wardrobe to offer me clothes every time I came home. Throughout my life I had been so envious of people who had that soft maternal figure, the best-friend-kind-of-mum you could turn to no matter what. But there are different ways to show love, and everyone has been conditioned to give and receive it in different forms.

My mum grew up in tough circumstances, leaving school after her O-Levels to help on the family farm. She had her own complicated relationship with her mother – my Nanna – who spent time away from home with postnatal depression following the arrival of both my mum and her brother. Back in those days, postnatal depression was not recognised and lots of people just thought she was insane, unfortunately. Mum trained as a hairdresser and worked tirelessly until she could buy her own salon. Just before I was sent away to school, my parents had bought a Bed & Breakfast (remember the three-poster bed!), so on top of being on her feet all day managing her business, she also worked a second job there every day too. She never stopped, as it was seven days a week, 365 days a year.

On top of coordinating three kids, she also made my dad his lunch every day. 'Otherwise, he wouldn't eat,' she'd always say. She was a traditional housewife and a career woman all in one. I have no doubt that she sacrificed so much of her own life to give us the kind of upbringing she never had. I owe her so much.

And yet I always craved tenderness. I was a child desperate for physical affection and verbal reassurance. I have memories of trying to hug my mum, only for her to tell me to get off her because she didn't like cuddles. I definitely grew up longing for affection and struggling with the rejection of not receiving it. I'd often lock myself in the toilet or run away and hide behind trees, just to get attention. And when I didn't get it, I assumed it was because I wasn't lovable. That belief rooted itself deep. I really did grow up believing that she didn't love me. I have vivid memories of driving to school with my dad as a thirteen-year-old and asking him why Mum hated me so much. 'She doesn't, man!' he said, quickly shutting the conversation down. I'm sure it drove them mad, this constant need for parental validation, but that sense that I was never enough still causes me pain, even though I have learned to be more rational about it. I know now that my parents did love me but they showed it in different ways, like working their socks off to make sure we were provided for. What is for sure is that, not finding it at home, I began looking for validation elsewhere.

I wouldn't experience affection until boys discovered me as a teenager, and, by that point, I was a terrible judge of what was and wasn't genuine. I started to chase people who would give me scraps of affection and called it connection. If someone was emotionally unavailable, I'd try even harder to prove I was worthy. I thought love would come from 'fixing' someone – like if I could just love them enough, they'd finally see my worth and love me back. It was like emotional labour in exchange for crumbs.

Once, while I was crying over a guy who had love-bombed me and then disappeared, my friend Francesca said something I'll never forget: 'Ashley, you don't love him. You just want him.' She went on, 'It's like when you wanted a Barbie doll as a kid. You don't want *him*; you want what he represents. You're confusing desire with love. How can you possibly *love* someone you hardly know, especially when what you *do* know of him makes you feel terrible about yourself?'

She had a point. I'd built whole romantic narratives around men I barely knew. I'd imagined futures with people who hadn't even shown up in the present. I'd romanticised poor behaviour and projected fantasies onto strangers. I thought I was chasing love, but I was chasing validation.

And then there were the red flags I ignored. At school, 'red flag' wasn't a concept. I didn't realise that misogyny, emotional unavailability or inconsistent behaviour were signs to run. I thought they were signs I needed to love harder. I thought I was *chosen* to be the one who changed them. Now I see it differently. Now I'm fluent in red flags.

If someone says, 'My ex was crazy,' that's not a warning about her – it's a warning about *him*.

If someone says, 'You're not like other girls,' I no longer hear it as a compliment. I hear it as a confession: he doesn't respect women.

If someone says, 'Don't be so sensitive,' what they mean is, 'I don't want to be held accountable.'

And here's what I wish I'd known sooner: if someone ghosts you, that *is* the closure. If they don't message you back, if they disappear, if they stop trying – you don't need more information. Their silence says enough. Write the long

WhatsApp message if you need to but send it to a friend. Or write it in your notes app and then delete it. Don't give them the satisfaction of another second of your energy. You don't need someone else to see your worth for it to exist.

Understanding my attachment style, my childhood and my old patterns didn't just help me become a better dater, it helped me become a better friend to myself. I no longer needed someone to pick me to feel complete. I no longer felt like love was something I had to earn through performance, sacrifice or perfection. That shift changed everything. I stopped chasing people who didn't see me. I stopped mistaking chaos for chemistry. I stopped accepting crumbs and calling it a feast. Because when you start to learn what real love looks like – safe, calm, steady – you stop craving the storm.

34.
Girlfriend Material

The problem with decentring men was I got so good at life without them that I was scared to let them back in. Between the ages of thirty-one and thirty-three, I had a truly amazing time. I'd finally learned to be comfortable on my own. I could travel whenever I wanted and spend time doing what I loved with the people I loved. Most weekends I would host big, fancy dinner parties in my flat with women – some friends and some from the industry that I loved and respected. I loved bringing women together. It felt like sisterhood.

Of course, there were moments when I felt lonely – like lying hungover on the sofa on weekend mornings, wishing I had someone to cuddle me and make me a bacon sandwich. But, overall, I was content and had regained so much confidence. You've seen how low that confidence had got to at points, and while there were still chinks in my armour, I was a different woman to the one who had boarded that plane to Mexico just a couple of years before.

As I celebrated my thirty-third birthday, I slowly realised that I was really ready to meet someone, and I felt I'd finally learned the skills to date in a healthy way. The problem was, whoever said there are plenty of fish in the sea clearly hadn't dated in the 2010s. I can tell you for sure that the sea had been chronically overfished, polluted, and was full of commitment-phobes.

I'd learned enough to know that I didn't want to date anyone in my industry, and that after-dark settings were not the ideal place to meet the love of your life. I didn't want men approaching me when I was DJing or when I was out with friends. I wasn't into scoping the club for hot guys, as it just wasn't my vibe. So that left me with the option of online dating.

I'll be honest – I was dubious. Maybe it was the old-school part of me, but I couldn't find the idea of connecting with strangers on the internet aspirational. On the other hand, unless Mr Perfect fell out of a plane and landed on my patio, I wasn't going to find him any other way. Initially, I downloaded a popular celebrity dating app that had been featured a lot in the press, but, honestly, I really didn't see the appeal. Half the people on it lived in America or Australia and were only in the UK temporarily. We all know what they were likely looking for, and it didn't end in 'happily ever after'. At one point, I matched with a Jonas brother (among a few other global superstars), but I ended up deleting the app and trying another one.

I can't tell you how many gym selfies I had to swipe past, how many immediately sexual conversations I had to block, and how many horrendous icks I encountered. I was also really nervous about meeting a total stranger from the internet. I had to really talk myself into taking the first step. 'See it as an interview,' someone suggested. 'You're both just figuring out if there's compatibility.' I decided to also use it as an opportunity to test my new skills as a red-flag spotter, boundary creator and avoidant-attachment escaper.

The first date I went on was at a fancy bar in central

London. We were having drinks and getting on when, out of the blue, he asked me what I thought of Binky and Spencer. Oh no! For the record, I wouldn't have minded discussing *Made in Chelsea* – it was more the fact that he'd never mentioned knowing anything about my background at any point in the previous two hours. It just felt strange and took me by surprise. There was no second date.

Date number two was with a guy I got on relatively well with. We ended up going on a couple more casual dates, and I even invited him out with my friends. We all went back to mine, and that's when he told me he was allergic to cats and didn't like dogs. By this point, I had three cats *and* a dog. There was no way it was going to work. I told him that – politely, of course. 'I can take antihistamines,' he said. What, forever?!

Date number three was Tommy.

The real story is that I'd got my wires crossed and hadn't realised it was actually a date. We'd started chatting after spotting each other on a dating app, but we already knew each other from Abercrombie & Fitch, back in the day. I'd actually left before Tommy started, but we'd been introduced through mutual friends at the store and used to bump into each other in random places. He was always with his very beautiful ex-girlfriend, and I thought they were such a hot couple that I never considered him as an individual (sorry, Tommy).

When we started chatting on Hinge, I assumed it was just two people catching up as friends. When he asked if I fancied continuing the chat over a roast dinner, I thought, why not? I'd firmly friend-zoned him in my mind. Sunday came around, and I'd already ended up eating (a full roast) at a friend's house. So, when 4 p.m. chimed and Tommy text to say he was outside the tube station, I thought, *shit*. I didn't have the heart to tell him I'd already had my lunch, so I geared myself up for round two. Hanging out with him felt natural and easy, and the conversation just flowed — probably because I hadn't considered it a romantic thing at all.

We still laugh about what happened next, and I really must stress: I *truly* wasn't aware I was on a date. I'd just done this big clothing campaign, and some of the images were on billboards around London. It was the first time anything like that had happened in my career, and it felt huge! I'd clocked that one billboard was only ten minutes away, so I asked Tommy if he'd come take some pics of me in front of it for the 'gram. I DIE at the idea that Tommy thought this was me trying to impress him. On my life, I would *never* have asked that of anyone I fancied. The cringe!

Anyway, underneath my own giant billboard (lol), Tommy leant in to kiss me — and the rest, as they say, is history.

I don't usually kiss on the first date — especially when I don't even know it's a date! I still don't know how he got away with it, but he was obviously charming and handsome, and my head was, I admit, turned. When he got home, he text to say what a nice time he'd had. Nothing gushing — just straightforward. My red-flag radar didn't flash once. There was absolutely nothing that set off my nervous system. That is *exactly* how it should feel.

With Tommy, all the things I had taught myself came easy. I didn't have to enforce strong boundaries because he never tried to intentionally push them. And because I didn't allow my brain to put him on a pedestal — I constantly reminded myself that I didn't really know him — it also meant I wasn't hugely invested in the outcome of our story. That was a first for me. There was no, *how should I act so he sees my worth?* There was just *this is who I am, and this is what I expect*. It was a major mindset shift. It meant I didn't disregard my own needs, and I didn't let the worry of being labelled crazy be prioritised above my own boundaries.

One of my non-negotiables at that point was that I only wanted to date someone who was looking for a relationship. Not necessarily with me, but in general. I was seeking someone who was actually in the market for a partnership. I wanted to know what he was looking for, and I didn't leave it to guesswork – I just asked him.

I also didn't want to end up in a physical relationship before confirming he wasn't sleeping with – or sexting – anyone else. No judgement if that works for you, but it wasn't for me. I'd been in so many situations with exes where really sketchy things had happened – crossovers, cheating – and I was just done. In the past, I'd entered sexual relationships hoping that men weren't seeing anyone else, but too scared to ask in case it made me seem 'too keen'.

'You're my boyfriend now,' I said to him after a few weeks. 'Umm, news to me,' Tommy replied. 'Well, you are. We've got to the point where if you were to message or date anyone else, I'd have to stop talking to you. So, you can call it what you want, but for all intents and purposes, you're my boyfriend. It's up to you if you want me to be your girlfriend,' I replied casually. Like I said, I'd rather be seen as crazy than be taken advantage of.

Tommy always said he was fascinated by my directness and that it was one of the things that attracted him to me. That's so funny to me, because this was the first time I'd ever been this direct with a man. But he didn't want to play games either. I said I'd rather date each other exclusively, know where we stood, and let it last a month, than play some long-drawn-out game that might technically last longer but was already over before it started. The stakes were really low for me – if it all turned to dust, I knew I'd be fine. That's the superpower of single joy: knowing you're okay on your own.

We met on 1 December 2019, and by the end of that month, I'd invited him to go to Finland with me for a few days in January. 'Let's just have adventures for as long as we like each other,' I said. I wasn't pretending or being the cool girl, I was just confident in myself. I knew what I wanted, and I wasn't going to live or die depending on whether this man decided he liked me or not. On 31 December 2019, he asked me to be his girlfriend. It's amazing how simple it can be when two people are emotionally available and looking for the same thing.

As excited as we were about each other, we also lived very independent lives. We saw each other twice a week. We were just enjoying getting to know each other, and I was still deeply invested in all the other amazing parts of the life I'd built. I wasn't letting anything else fall by the wayside. This was my first relationship in six years, and it took a lot of getting used to because I'd become so used to suiting myself.

I had changed a lot. I was no longer seeking a co-dependent relationship where I needed a 'best friend' (I already had my best friends). I wasn't looking for my 'other half' because I knew I was already complete on my own. We're not these half-humans walking around waiting to be tessellated into a missing piece of a jigsaw puzzle.

I told Tommy that I never wanted to get married, and that I didn't even want to move in together. Maybe, if things progressed, we could think about getting flats in the same area, or even houses on the same street. I wasn't being frosty or playing hard to get. I'd just changed how I pictured my happy ending, and it no longer involved me in a white dress and veil, being swept over the threshold into a marital home.

BALL AND CHAIN
bɔːl ənd tʃeɪn
noun

a slang term – often used jokingly – to describe a wife or long-term female partner as a burden, restriction or source of lost freedom for a man. It frames marriage or commitment not as a mutual partnership but as something that traps men and kills their spontaneity or masculinity. The woman becomes the obstacle to fun, adventure or autonomy.

Male equivalent: There is no real male equivalent. We don't have a common phrase that frames husbands or male partners as deadweight or freedom-killers. In fact, men are rarely portrayed as the problem in a relationship in the same jokey, cultural shorthand. Instead, commitment is often seen as something women crave and men tolerate. *Ball and chain* reflects the sexist cultural script that assumes men are naturally independent and adventurous, while women are clingy, limiting and domestic. It reduces women to the role of fun-suppressor and positions men as the victims of female attachment.

35.
Happily Never After

I don't want to get married. It's one of the opinions I find hardest to share – not because I doubt it, but because I know I'm in the minority, and I never want it to sound like a criticism.

So, I want to caveat this chapter and say, if you're someone who dreams of getting married, I am truly happy for you, and I really hope you have the wedding of your dreams. I'll be there on your big day, having a ball, celebrating you, because I love seeing people do what makes them happy. Marriage can be amazing! I don't think it's anti-feminist or anti-progressive to get married, even if you stick to tradition. The beauty of it is in the *choice*. We are all products of a patriarchal society, and we are all walking contradictions – I know I am. I get Botox while recognising that anti-ageing is based on toxic patriarchal standards. We're also allowed to change our minds a thousand times, and that's okay too. I have lots of friends who got married – especially queer friends – who see it as a chance to rewrite history. To celebrate societal progress and to have their love recognised like everyone else's. That's a beautiful thing, and I am here for it. So, if you dream of a white wedding, I don't judge you and I will be delighted for you if and when it happens.

However, when it comes to my own aspirations, I am to

marriage what the Grinch is to Christmas. I had always assumed I'd get hitched; remember my invisible timeline with my ex? Engaged after university, married by twenty-six. I had never given much actual consideration to marriage, but assumed that that's just what happens when you're a grown-up and you meet someone and fall in love. It was the only 'happily ever after' I thought existed. But being single for so long made me question the status quo. I started to really scrutinise the institution and its traditions, and I realised that maybe it just wasn't for me.

Today there are no maybes. I know I don't want to get married. Not in a vague, maybe-one-day kind of way. I know in a clear, steady, deep-in-my-bones kind of way. I've interrogated it, sat with it, and turned it over in my mind again and again. And every time I come back to the same answer: it's not for me. And yet – I still feel grief about it. Or maybe confusion. Not because I doubt my decision, but because it's strange to feel so out of step with the world around me. Marriage is celebrated, longed for, obsessed over. It's the grand finale of every rom com, the social milestone that earns applause, the moment people post about with glittery captions and diamond emojis. It's treated as both a personal triumph and cultural checkpoint. People light up when it's on the horizon. And I . . . don't. What do you do with that? I often wish I could understand the hype, and sometimes feel like I am missing out on so much excitement. And I've really *really* tried to get it.

From the outside, marriage can look like love, security and celebration, but there is another side. When you peel back the glossy layers of Pinterest boards and diamond ring ads, you'll find an institution with deep patriarchal roots. For centuries, marriage wasn't about love – it was about ownership. Dowries, arranged marriages and strategic alliances were the norm. A woman's value lay in her virginity and fertility; her husband gained rights to her body, labour and even her children. She gained a home, social legitimacy and protection – not from him, but from other men. But she didn't get any power, even over her own body.

Marriage was never a partnership of equals; it was a hierarchy. The man led; the woman followed. And for centuries in Britain, the law upheld this imbalance under the legal doctrine of *coverture*. A woman lost her legal identity the moment she married, becoming one person with her husband in the eyes of the law – *his person, not hers*. It's why so many letters still address married couples as Mr and Mrs [insert man's name]. He had authority over her body, her property, even her freedom of movement. She couldn't own assets, enter contracts or have custody of her own children. Marriage didn't just unite two people – it erased one of them. As we've covered earlier, according to coverture, it wasn't possible for a husband to rape his lawful wife because a woman had given permanent sexual consent once she married and she couldn't take it back. Ever.

> *The husband cannot be guilty of a rape committed by himself upon his lawful wife, for by their mutual matrimonial consent and contract the wife hath given herself up in this kind unto her husband, which she cannot retract.*
>
> —Jurist Sir Matthew Hale, 1736

A wedding was a transaction, a transfer of ownership from one man to another. That's why we still talk about 'giving the bride away'. Everyone seems to love the father walking the bride down the aisle, and it's always framed as a sweet and sentimental moment, and if you just take it at face value, it can be exactly that. And seeing how proud and elated my dad was to walk my sister down the aisle on her wedding day, who am I to tell anyone not to enjoy that moment? I said to my sister that I was so glad she'd chosen a traditional wedding, so my dad got to have that moment. But through my eyes? I see a ritual that symbolically transfers ownership from one man to another. And I can't help wondering: why are we still acting this out in the 2020s? My dad doesn't own me, and nor would any husband. So why are we cosplaying patriarchal history?

This is also why, traditionally, it's the bride's family who is expected to foot the bill. By 'marrying off' a daughter and receiving a dowry (a financial gift or payment given to the groom or his family), a family could gain a significant influx of cash, so paying for the wedding was seen as part of the deal. The same goes for the groom asking the bride's father for permission to marry her. I've always found it strange that the decision is still framed as something that needs another man's blessing. Isn't *her* 'yes' enough? Again, it's another tradition that came from needing a father's consent to proceed with a marriage because he had authority over the family's alliances, finances and reputation. A suitor needed approval because the daughter was part of a broader transaction. These days, the idea that *not* asking a father is somehow disrespectful or poor manners is just wild to me. Even if the intention is sweet, the roots are tangled in the belief that a woman is to be handed over, not that she's an autonomous adult making her own choice.

I hope you're starting to understand why I find so much of this depressing, and why so much of it gives me the patriarchal ick.

Even today, some women are still asked to promise to 'obey' their soon-to-be-husbands in traditional wedding vows, while grooms are only expected to love and cherish. That difference speaks volumes about the role women were expected to play within the historical structure of marriage. Much of this comes from religious teachings, which positioned the husband as the 'head of the household' and the wife as the obedient supporter: *'Wives, submit yourselves unto your own husbands, as unto the Lord. For the husband is the head of the wife . . .'* Ephesians 5:22–24. It wasn't actually until 1973 that the Anglican Church began quietly allowing couples to remove the word 'obey' from the script. Although Queen Elizabeth II left it out of her wedding vows to Prince Philip in 1947. A power move, but then again, she *was* Her Royal Highness.

While we might not be forced to promise to 'obey' our husbands anymore, male voices still dominate wedding speeches at traditional weddings. We hear speeches from the father of the bride, the best man and the groom, but women's voices are conspicuously absent. WHY DOES NO ONE WANT TO HEAR FROM ANY OF THE WOMEN? The best man's speech is often particularly puke-inducing with its wink-wink references to the groom's wild past, drunken antics and sexual conquests. I can't help but think how horrendously inappropriate this is as the groom sits next to his silent bride dressed in virginal white. I also wonder how the room would react if the roles were reversed and bridesmaids stood up to share stories of the bride's past sexual escapades, told with the same cheeky charm. Now *that* is a wedding I'd love to attend!

See, I told you I'm the Grinch! That's why weddings make me feel so . . . conflicted. Not because I don't love *love*, I still very much do. But because of what I can't ignore.

There are still so many wedding traditions that are accepted as norms today that are rooted in the restriction of women's freedoms and I find that so problematic. Let's take the white dress. Wearing white became a bridal tradition after Queen Victoria wore a white gown at her wedding in 1840. Before this point, brides just wore the best dress in their wardrobe, often brightly coloured. For the Queen, a white dress was a symbol of wealth as very few people could afford to buy a dress they'd only wear once. Especially, a white one given the filthy streets of nineteenth-century England. Over time, white came to symbolise virginity and purity. It was a not-so-subtle way of announcing that the bride was untouched, and therefore *worthy*.

That's the part I can't shake: the way it ties a woman's value to whether or not her body has been 'used'. As if wearing white is a reward for staying small, quiet and clean. The implication that female sexual desire makes us dirty makes me never want to wear a white dress again.

Let's move onto the bling! Now don't get me wrong, I LOVE a ring, especially a big fat diamond one. The bigger the better for me! But something about wearing a public declaration of someone's financial commitment – instead of mutual love – feels odd. Engagement rings originated as a public claim and clear signal that a woman was no longer on the market, as if we were chattels to be bought and sold to the highest bidder. Men didn't wear rings because, of course, they didn't need proof of ownership. While things have unquestionably evolved, many married men still refuse to wear wedding rings, and wearing one is even considered frightfully common in aristocratic circles. I found it interesting that, at the King's Coronation, neither King Charles, Prince William nor the Duke of Edinburgh wore wedding rings, but Prince Harry did. The late Prince Philip never wore one, and nor do Boris Johnson or Donald Trump. Read into that what you will!

Even when you break down weddings to the most granular

level, a lot of the traditions are just . . . odd. Like the bouquet toss! Nothing makes me run further than the moment when all the unmarried women gather round to catch the bouquet in the hope that they will be next to be picked. Like the aliens in *Toy Story* hoping to be chosen by their new master. The only thing that makes it worse is the faces of the men looking on in feigned terror at the thought of having to settle down with their own 'ball and chain'.

It's strange, isn't it, how commitment and marriage are framed as aspirational for women, while for men they're often portrayed as something to be avoided or reluctantly agreed to. As little girls, we're told fairy tales that end with a wedding, and encouraged to dream of our own 'special day' — long before we've even figured out what we want in life, let alone in a partner. The language around marriage is revealing too: women are 'chosen', 'wife material', 'waiting for the one'. It's always about being *picked*, not about *choosing*. Meanwhile, men are often portrayed as *losing* something in marriage: their freedom, their fun, their independence. Commitment is framed as a reluctant sacrifice, the stag being the 'last night of freedom'. But when you look at the deal on paper, to me this feels like societal gaslighting. Men are arguably getting the better end of the bargain, at least in relationships that follow traditional gender roles. A husband gains a live-in cook, cleaner, maid, nanny, therapist, and potential vessel for their future heir — all for free. A wife, on the other hand, will take on more unpaid labour[28] and will find that the pressure and stress of family life disproportionately lies on her shoulders. This is all statistically true. And yet we are still sold the myth that *we* are the lucky ones if we get asked. Convincing women that a contract in which they shoulder most of the invisible, unpaid labour is a prize — while men are positioned as the reluctant givers of this 'gift' of commitment – has to be the greatest PR stunt of all time. The devil works hard, but the patriarchal PR machine works harder.

It should be men rugby tackling each other for that bouquet, because THE AUDACITY. We're raised to believe that marriage is our reward for being pleasing enough. That it's something to hope for, to wait for. That if no one asks us, we've failed or not played our cards properly.

Marriage was designed to benefit men, and yet *we're* often the ones driving the fantasy. All while giving up our names and with the expectation that our babies take the man's name even though they are nearly all made inside *our* bodies. What in the name of successful societal gaslighting is that?

It's a hard no from me.

I understand that it can be tricky to empathise with feelings that sit so far out of the norm, but I do find it infuriating that people either assume I'm already married to Tommy or that he just hasn't asked me yet. A journalist recently asked if I thought Tommy might 'pop the question' soon.

'I hope not,' I replied, to her obvious horror.

For me, marriage isn't the problem. The expectation that it defines us is. If marriage works for you, brilliant. But I refuse to be boxed into someone else's idea of 'happily ever after'. I don't want to be chosen, I want to choose for myself.

36.
Bride and Prejudice?

Despite my views on marriage, I had fallen – hook, line and sinker – for Tommy. Love stories don't always need a ring and a white dress to be valid. It's okay to love deeply without conforming to societal and religious expectations even if others don't understand it. And I love Tommy.

He is a kind and insanely attractive man who is always upfront and honest. He always calls out poor behaviour, stands up for women, and is a man of true integrity. After six years of singlehood and thinking maybe there were no 'good men' out there, something I know many of you will relate to, it turns out some do exist. There are loyal ones you don't have to lose sleep over, worrying whether they will cheat. Ones who will hold your hand through the worst days of your life. Ones that will make you laugh rather than cry. They are out there, they just hide really *really* well.

It brings me back to all those fish in the sea. I always say Tommy is my coelacanth – bear with me for the niche reference! A coelacanth is an ancient fish so rare it was thought to be extinct for millions of years, until it was rediscovered in 1938. That's literally how it felt to find a good and emotionally available man. So instead of telling people there are plenty of fish out there, maybe we should say: if you look hard enough, you might just be lucky enough to find a coelacanth. Good ones are scarce, but they exist. So don't throw your line down for a common carp, no matter how dark the ocean feels, and try to enjoy fishing – or not fishing – while you wait.

So how do I describe my love story outside of the well-trodden path of traditional marriage? Once you strip it all back, what is left? For me, the answer is love.

The idea that love would even be a factor in our relationships is actually relatively new, only a few hundred years old at best. It wasn't really until the eighteenth and early nineteenth centuries that romantic love started to elbow its way into the narrative, and, even then, it was more of a theory than a reality for most. Think of Jane Austen's novels, full of the tension between marrying for love and marrying to survive. Charlotte Lucas in *Pride and Prejudice* doesn't say yes to Mr Collins because she's in love, she says yes because she has no other option. As a woman without her own fortune, love was a luxury she couldn't afford.

We had to wait until the early twentieth century for arranged marriages and dowries to fade from everyday Western culture, particularly among working- and middle-class families. The radical shift that women might actually have a say in who they married was sparked by industrialisation and the women's movement, but it wasn't until the 1960s and 70s that love-based marriage became the new standard. Feminists fought for reproductive rights, financial autonomy, the right to divorce and equal footing in relationships. For the first time in modern history, women were allowed to *choose* marriage, and just as importantly, *choose* to leave it without being ruined in the process.

'Happily ever after' may have successfully rebranded marriage, but how do we really know we'll love the same person forever? Is that a realistic expectation to have? I always say to Tommy that I choose him every day. And loving him also means being willing to let him go, should the time come when I'm no longer the person who makes him happy, or vice versa. How can we possibly know at thirty-eight what will make us happy at seventy-four? Doesn't seventy-four-year-old me, and/or seventy-four-year-old Tommy, deserve to feel in love, fulfilled and free, just as much as we do now?

Despite all of the above, I recognise marriage still offers legal and financial protection. 'I've found a positive reason to get married,' I once said to Tommy, 'it offers financial security if one of us dies.' 'How romantic!' he replied. See, at the start of our relationship, Tommy couldn't quite understand why I didn't want to get married. He'd never really thought about it himself; he just saw it as a natural next step when you love someone and want to build a life with them. I once asked him to pitch me the reasons he wanted to get married so I could try to understand it and get on board. 'A pitch?' he laughed. 'You want me to pitch marriage to you? Don't worry about it.'

I should add that money expert (and life guru) Martin Lewis once told me on *This Morning* that the most financially savvy thing any woman could do was to get married – especially if there were children involved. I told him I'd rather fight the system and make it fair so we didn't have to, and in reply he warned me I could pay dearly for that principle.

My financial advisor recently gave me the same advice, not only to protect Tommy and myself, but also our children. In the UK, if you're married and your partner dies, you automatically inherit anything you own jointly. But if you're unmarried, it depends how your assets are held, and anything left to you can be taxed at up to 40 per cent, even if you're named in the will. If you're not named, the estate bypasses you entirely and goes into a trust for the children until they're eighteen.

If you own a house together, you may be forced to sell it to release your children's share. That's why we hear stories of unmarried mothers losing their family homes. When you're married, you don't have to think about any of that.

When I lay it out, even I start to question my stubbornness. Marriage makes sense. If I'd given up my career to provide childcare and home support so that my husband could work, I think I'd feel differently. If that is you, I would even advise you to get married. Marriage acts as an insurance policy for women who step away from their own careers to support their family and take on unpaid domestic and childcare labour. Women should absolutely make smart legal and financial decisions to protect themselves in case a relationship breaks down. If you've sacrificed your job, your income, your time and your pension so that your partner can build his career and bring in the money, then it should be impossible for him to walk away and leave you with nothing but the bare minimum in child maintenance.

Yet we still cling to the idea that women 'take half' if a marriage ends, as if they've won some unfair prize. What's rarely acknowledged is that many have given far more than half. They've given up their financial independence, their career progression, their security in old age. They've taken on all the invisible, unpaid work that makes their partner's success possible. So next time you hear someone say a woman has 'taken him to the cleaners', maybe question if that's true. Is she really a gold digger, or did she just get her fair share?

There are still very real barriers for women like me – women who have children, who live in committed relationships, but who simply don't want to be legally partnered. All I want is to *exist* as an unmarried woman with the same protections and without people assuming my partner just hasn't asked me yet. Or that, when I meet the *right* person, I'll change my mind. It's insulting to imply that, if I *really* loved Tommy, I'd be prepared to overlook the history of oppression tied up in marriage.

But I also recognise what a privilege it is to be able to choose not to marry. A choice that so many of our ancestors didn't get and a choice that many women around the world still don't have. I can own my own home, live with my partner as an unwed woman, and my children can exist without being considered 'illegitimate'. And that choice is thanks to feminism.

So if you *choose* to get married, I am delighted for you. Commitment *can* be beautiful, but only when it's mutual, equitable and freely entered into, not when it's expected of women and optional for men. For me, I choose 'happily *never* after'. I choose personal rebellion and cultural reimagining. Dare I say I even revel in my status as an unwed mother as a tribute to all the women who came before me who were shamed and punished. I am not saying I want you to reconsider marriage, but I hope it encourages you to at least ask if marriage is truly your story, or just society's.

Now I just need the world to catch up and stop assuming Tommy is my husband!

I do sometimes feel bad for Tommy. I know he would have loved a wedding, even if he understands my views about it. But he knew what he was signing up for. From day one, I told him I didn't even envisage myself living with a man. It might sound silly, but after being by myself for so long, I honestly couldn't imagine sharing my pink, feminine flat with a man. And, in any case, where would all his stuff go? Tommy loves football and I couldn't imagine my TV being taken over with sport. The sound of men's football still irritates me, to be fair.

But, as it turned out, once he moved in – unofficially – he would never leave.

On 23 March 2020, Prime Minister Boris Johnson announced the UK's first national lockdown in response to the Covid-19 pandemic. That same evening, I told Tommy he had to go back to his own flat. 'We don't know how long this will go on for!' I insisted. 'Well, that's sort of why I thought I'd stay here,' he replied gently. After a few hours of sitting with the guilt and thinking it over, I realised that maybe – just maybe – I was being a little stubborn. Because, despite my fierce independence, my pink sofa, and my years of solo resilience, the truth was clear: I was in love with Tommy.

So, I clung on to my coelacanth and, just ten months later, Tommy and I were still living together . . . with our newborn baby. Life really can change in the blink of an eye, and you just cannot predict wtf is going to happen next. I'm so glad Tommy had been up for that adventure in Finland with me after only four weeks of dating, otherwise we'd have never travelled abroad together before we became parents!

So, I didn't get 'the rock', but I got something better: freedom, love, and a family I chose on my own terms. Oh, and I bought myself a ring. I wear it every day as a reminder of my choices. The ring features my daughter's birthstone cut in a heart shape. Surrounding the heart are my own birthstones: diamonds. It's a symbol of my independence – a vintage ring, which meant it once belonged to one of the women who came before me. Maybe for her it was a sign of ownership. But for me it's a talisman of freedom. If that isn't a 'happily ever after', I don't know what is.

MOTHERHOOD

MUMSY

ˈmʌm.zi
adjective

a patronising term used to describe a woman as frumpy or overly domestic. The insinuation that mothers are unfashionable alludes to the loss of identity, sexuality or relevance in favour of practicality, comfort or caregiving. A *mumsy* woman is rarely seen as powerful or desirable, just dependable, gentle and a bit dull.

Male equivalent: There's no true male equivalent, unless of course you want to try and say 'dadsy' – but you'll probably be the first one to go there. Fathers aren't typically reduced to stereotypes that imply they've let themselves go or become uncool by embracing parenthood. In fact, *dad* aesthetics, like 'dad bod' or 'dad jokes', are often treated with affection or humour, not scorn. *Mumsy* reflects how unforgiving we are when women no longer prioritise being desirable. It's yet another way language punishes women for growing older, choosing comfort or devoting themselves to others.

37.
The Mother of All Labels

Motherhood was *not* in my five-year plan. Or even my ten-year plan. In fact, I didn't want to be a mum. I thought maternal instinct was something for other women – something that had skipped me – and I suppose I saw motherhood as a kind of anti-feminist act. A vanishing of self. I didn't want to lose my freedom, my body, my identity. I'd spent so much of my life trying to carve out space for myself, and I wasn't ready to give it up. But life doesn't always follow the script. Sometimes it throws you a plot twist.

I didn't get pregnant intentionally – it was very much not planned. It still feels taboo to say that out loud. A sensible adult, especially a 'lady', is supposed to do things in the 'right' order: be in a long-term relationship, get married, and only then make a conscious decision to have a baby. An unexpected pregnancy is still framed as the result of some *silly girl* who got herself knocked up, or a *careless woman* who didn't organise her birth control. But here's what comforts me: 45 per cent of pregnancies in England are unplanned[29] at the time of conception. That's nearly half. So, clearly, it's not just me.

When you're honest about having an unplanned pregnancy, people love to warn you that your child might grow up feeling unwanted, or like a mistake. I find that such a strange attitude. Statistically, many of our children will one day find themselves in the same position. Would I ever resent my parents for telling me I was unplanned? Not unless they also told me they regretted going through with it.

We're lucky to live in a time where we have a choice – and we have abortion rights to thank for that. Whether or not a pregnancy was planned becomes irrelevant once the decision is made. What matters is that it was your decision.

As a teenager, I assumed I'd have kids by twenty-seven, because that's what you naturally do when you're older, right? But, by my early thirties, I'd started to think I might never want to become a parent. As the birthdays came and went, and I had the space to really think about it, I realised I might not be a natural mum. When I met Tommy, I told him straight: if having children was a dealbreaker, he should probably date someone else. But fate had different plans – the pandemic hit, and neither of us had time to mull it over.

The truth is, I didn't feel a deep maternal pull or a burning desire to become a mum. Some women know they want to be mothers their whole lives. I know plenty of women who've always felt it was what they were naturally born to do. Others, like me, simply do not. I kept waiting for that biological pulse people talked about, that light-switch moment when instinct kicks in and everything makes sense. I'm here to tell you that, for me, it never happened.

I didn't grow up around children. I did work as an au pair briefly in my early twenties, but from twenty-one to thirty-one, I lived a life entirely detached from anyone under the age of eighteen. I had no personal connection to a single child. And as I started to properly understand how much motherhood impacted women's lives, I came to a pretty firm conclusion: kids would derail my career and limit my freedom. I know I'm not alone in thinking that. Plenty of us have looked at exhausted friends stretched thin, drowning in plastic toys and the mental load, and thought – yeah, that's not for me.

The idea of women having maternal instincts is sold as universal and innate. If it doesn't hit you like a truck, you assume you don't have 'it'. But maternal feelings are diverse and can be influenced by lots of different factors. You might long for a baby but feel terrified of the version of motherhood you've seen – a lonely mum stuck at home alone, pacing the house with one eye on the monitor and a mug of cold coffee in hand. Fear can muffle desire, even when it's instinctual.

So, I told myself I wasn't maternal. How could I be? I practically ran out of the door after seeing friends with their babies and their overstimulating and noisy, plastic-covered homes. But during my deep dive into psychology in my late twenties and early thirties, I learned about limiting beliefs – these are the subjective ideas we hold about ourselves and the world that shape our experience. One of my limiting beliefs was that I wasn't maternal. I'd convinced myself I just didn't possess that gene.

It was quite the shock when my babies were born and I had an immediate, instinctive connection to them. I knew exactly what to do. For all the things that annihilated my mental health after becoming a mum, that maternal bond was never one of them. I'd been completely wrong about myself.

I knew I was pregnant almost the minute I conceived because my boobs hurt so much. *Uh-oh.*

Tommy and I had just got together and were still under the six-month mark. I was convinced that I didn't want to live with a man, didn't want to get married, and didn't want kids. My career was finally going from strength to strength, and I felt confident and happy after nearly twenty years of having it bashed out of me. Oh yeah, and it also felt like we were living in a zombie apocalypse as we were sanitising our packages before bringing them into the house, navigating food and loo-paper shortages, and watching reports of bodies piling up in New York. Let's just say 'baby' was not on my bingo card.

Because we were only allowed to leave the house for a quick walk around the park, I had to order the pregnancy tests online and wait for them to arrive. When they did, I took three in a row. Each one was positive. *Shit*, I thought. *What was Tommy going to think?*

I rang my friend immediately to ask what to do. 'I can't have this baby, I'm too young!' She laughed out loud. 'Ashley, there are a million reasons why you might not be in the right place to have a baby, but you're thirty-four. The "I'm too young to be a mother" ship has sailed.' *How dare she!*

While I was still figuring out what to do, Tommy went to borrow a pair of tweezers and discovered all the pregnancy tests in my drawer. 'WHEN WERE YOU GOING TO TELL ME?!' he shouted.

I was petrified he'd be angry with me (because obviously it was my fault). Instead, he threw his arms around me. 'THIS IS AMAZING!' he said.

Is it? I thought. I don't know why his reaction surprised me; I think I'd always assumed men wouldn't want a baby. I suppose we've been socially conditioned to fear getting pregnant out of wedlock. His excitement was infectious, and I was so bowled over by the fact that he wanted to have a child with me. I do remember going through a thousand 'buts', though – 'but I'm a DJ!' and 'but I don't even like kids!' among them.

Very quickly thoughts of doing anything else but going ahead with the pregnancy evaporated. *How bad could it really be?* Everyone had spent the last six years telling me how I'd regret not having kids – that I was making a big mistake choosing to be child-free. So surely it was the right thing to do?

It sounds strange now, given I'd never wanted kids, but it really did feel like fate. Like life had been waiting for this moment to bring it all together. Every heartbreak, every disappointment, every obstacle I'd overcome and the distance I had travelled to get to this point – both literally and metaphorically. It felt like destiny.

Once we'd wrapped our heads around our news, it felt amazing to have this ray of hope amid all the fear and uncertainty of the pandemic. We rang our parents, who, thankfully, we had both met in person just before lockdown. The first thing Tommy's mum said to me when I first met her was, 'Please, can you make me a nana?', so we had no doubt about how thrilled his parents would be. And they were.

My parents were a little more . . . surprised. Calling them, I felt like a sixteen-year-old girl again, having to tell them that I'd 'messed up'. I was so nervous that I made random small talk as Tommy nudged me. 'You're going to be grandparents!' I suddenly blurted.

'Your sister hasn't told us she's having a baby,' my dad said, confused. My sister was the only married sibling, after all. They are very traditional, and I think it simply hadn't occurred to them that their older, unmarried daughter might be the one calling with the baby news – especially since I'd always insisted I didn't want kids.

'Oh,' they said, slightly shell-shocked, 'who's the father?'

You can always rely on my dad's dry northern humour to break the ice.

But beneath the jokes, I wondered if they were worried about telling people they knew that I was having a baby with a man I'd just met. A well-meaning friend asked me if we were going to get married before the baby was here. *So that I am not a 'ruined woman', you mean,* I thought to myself – knowing she didn't intentionally mean to imply that. But that's what I would have been, not all that long ago.

Either way, it hit me: motherhood isn't just a personal shift. It comes with a whole set of new boxes I was now expected to climb into – and shrink myself to fit. Boxes I'd once mocked too.

And that's when I realised something uncomfortable: it wasn't just society that had absorbed these stereotypes about mums. I had, too.

38.
One of 'Those' Mums

If my journey into motherhood has taught me anything, it's how deeply my own internalised misogyny ran. I had proudly considered myself a feminist, yet I was horrendously prejudiced against mothers. I just hadn't noticed – not until there was no escaping my own narrow-minded attitudes.

I'll be honest: before I became a mother, I had no real idea what it entailed. I probably said things like 'enjoy your time off' to colleagues heading off on maternity leave, and I definitely gasped in horror at the thought of paternity leave. 'How ridiculous, men don't have babies!' I'd moan about how unfair it was that child-free women didn't get the equivalent of maternity leave, because 'we deserved time off too'. I saw my place in society as being at odds with a mother's – I was fighting the patriarchy; she was upholding it. I thought her gain was my loss.

The truth is I looked down on mums from a great height. I said I never wanted to look 'mumsy'. Even if I did have kids, I told myself, I wouldn't have 'mum friends', and I'd never wear frumpy 'mum' clothes – as if every other woman before me had suddenly decided to give up on fashion and start dressing conservatively in floral dresses and aprons like she was auditioning for *Little House on the Prairie*.

I proudly declared myself a 'career woman', which is why

I'd never had children. I believed those roles to be inherently incompatible without ever questioning why men never had to choose between fatherhood and a job. Without realising how insulting that was to all the career women who *had* given birth.

I was once sat next to a man in a bar in my early twenties (it was a group setting – I wasn't on a date!) and he suddenly said he had to go because his wife was 'nagging' him. I swore I'd never be like one of *those* boring older women (casual ageism plus sexism, lovely). Now, I look back and think: WHY WERE YOU IN A BAR WITH A BUNCH OF TWENTY-ONE-YEAR-OLDS, GARY? YOUR POOR WIFE HAS BEEN WITH THE KIDS ALL DAY. GO HOME AND SHARE SOME OF THE PARENTAL RESPONSIBILITIES!

I also told myself that, if I ever did have a child, I'd never be one of *those* mums who *only* talked about their kids. You know, the ones who give up their fulfilling lives and just post drivel online about weaning. 'NO ONE CARES, CAROL,' I'd scream internally, while uploading pictures of people I barely knew. Of course *that* was acceptable.

I once told my friend Jackie that I loved how she 'never talked about her kids' – not like all the other mums. Since having children myself, I issued her a full apology. She told me she liked hanging out with me because she got to feel like 'Jackie the woman' and not just 'Jackie the mum', which was the case with the rest of her life. That made me feel a little better, but the fact I said it at all – how dare I?

I was a proper dick. I'm really sorry.

But I wasn't born with these attitudes, I had been taught them. *We* are taught them. These weren't views I made up myself, they were part of a much bigger story we tell about motherhood. A story that shrinks women the moment they become mums. Society tells us that once we've had our babies, we're no longer sexy, no longer relevant, no longer powerful. We're expected to be selfless, invisible and grateful, while also being stylish, natural, slim and back at work with a smile. Easy!

Mums are either framed as frumpy and boring, or as irresponsible and selfish for wanting anything outside of their kids. The same culture that tells us motherhood is a woman's highest calling also laughs at us when we answer that call. We go from being women to 'just a mum' in a heartbeat. No wonder I didn't want to look 'mumsy'. The word itself is used as an insult. It's not just a style critique, it's a warning. Be careful. Don't become *her*. Don't lose your spark. Don't age. Don't become someone who exists solely in service of others. We learn early on that becoming a mum means disappearing. But now I know that mothers don't disappear, we're systematically erased. And it's time we stopped pretending that's inevitable.

I look back at that old judgemental version of myself and feel horrified. And I wonder why there's such a deep misunderstanding and disconnect around motherhood? Why mums are so often the butt of the joke, and why so much of what they do goes unseen and unappreciated – even by women who label themselves feminists. At the time, I suppose I believed feminism was about fighting against social norms and traditional milestones – marriage, pregnancy, motherhood. Within that context, becoming a mum felt like giving in to the very limitations that patriarchy had created for me simply because I was born female. But I was about to see everything through new eyes.

What I would soon realise was that motherhood sits right at the heart of so many feminist battles, and that by leaving mothers out of the conversation, we harm *all* women. Not just the ones who become mums. Because how we treat mothers reveals what we really think about women.

The mental load. The judgement. The isolation. The expectation to do it all and never complain. We speak about motherhood as if it's natural, instinctive, selfless and, in doing so, we devalue the labour of it. We fail to protect the women doing it and we make it harder for any woman to imagine herself in that role, especially if she's been taught that mums are boring, 'mumsy' or uncool.

Before becoming a mum, I thought I had feminism all figured out. But I was still carrying ideas that kept me judging other women and therefore serving the patriarchy. I accepted the negative narratives that are attached to the labels that come with motherhood, without questioning the systems that make it so difficult for them to thrive.

Motherhood cracked that open. And it would go on to change everything. Not just the way I saw mums. But the way I saw women. The way I saw power. The way I saw myself. And once I saw it, there was no going back.

39.
The Negative Nancys and the Just-You-Waits

It feels like the moment you tell the world you're having a baby, you invite unsolicited advice and judgement. It becomes almost instantly evident how much mums are pitted against each other. The running commentary about my bump and future child really took me by surprise. There is something about becoming pregnant that makes people suddenly decide to patronise you and treat you like a child. And the bigger your bump grows, the bigger the critique: 'Wow, your bump is enormous – good luck birthing that!', 'Whatever you do, make sure you get a C-section!', 'Should you be drinking caffeine?'

I like to call these people the 'Negative Nancys' and their gang of 'Just-You-Waits', because they seem to be permanently on call with negative, doom-laden comments.

> *Just you wait until you're not sleeping.*
> *Just you wait until they start teething.*
> *Just you wait until the tantrums.*
> *If you think it's hard being pregnant, just you wait until you have a newborn.*
> *You think having a newborn is hard, just you wait until you have a toddler!*

Instead of support, this constant scaremongering creates anxiety, steals joy from the present and plants seeds of self-doubt in women who are already navigating huge physical and emotional shifts. And it doesn't stop at pregnancy; they like to stick around for the whole motherhood journey.

> *You think juggling work and nursery is hard, just you wait until they're at school!*

These remarks rarely come from a place of empathy; more often than not people are just projecting their own difficult experiences in a very passive aggressive way. Some people might genuinely believe they're helping by sharing things they wish they'd been warned about, but the intention doesn't undo the impact. These comments can undermine someone's genuine feelings and can feel dismissive, condescending or even a bit smug, as though no one could possibly know what's coming or handle it well. And it's silly really, because my challenges won't necessarily be the same as yours.

Everyone's experience of motherhood is different. Our journeys are dependent on so many factors: our individual experiences, tolerances, circumstances, the networks around us, and most importantly the children themselves. Yes, there are hard parts. But there are also beautiful, empowering and funny parts. Giving out generalised 'just you wait' advice assumes everyone's experience will be the same, or that there's only one way to parent, which simply isn't true. Even between my two children, my experiences have been entirely different. What new mothers need is encouragement, space to feel how they feel, and the freedom to find their own rhythm, not a running commentary on everything that might go wrong.

I'll be honest and say I also struggled to bite my tongue at comments from first-time mums during my second pregnancy. I often felt triggered and had to resist the urge to 'just you wait' myself. 'I'm so tired today, all I've done is nap,' they'd say, and I'd think, *'Just you wait until you're pregnant and have a toddler. Naps are a luxury!'* Or when they'd announce they were never going to give their children plastic, or screen time, or white noise machines . . . *JUST YOU WAIT,* I'd think.

But I didn't say it. Because I remember what it felt like to hear those comments myself. I also remember the things I said when I was a first-time mum! We have to let people figure things out in their own time.

40.
Mum Wars

After birth, the judgement intensifies and there's a pressure to justify and defend every decision and instinct to yourself and others. Topics such as infant sleep and feeding have somehow become controversial and divisive, yet another impossible square you can't circle. No matter what you do, you can't win, and instead of focusing on your baby, it often feels like you're on a tightrope, with judgement waiting for you either side. You're judged for not breastfeeding at all, judged for using formula, judged for breastfeeding for too short a time, judged for breastfeeding for too long, and even judged for breastfeeding in public.

The consequence is that women torture themselves over dropping feeds or switching to formula. They feel like failures when their supply dips, or when their babies won't latch. Some mums hide bottles in public out of fear they'll be judged for not breastfeeding, while others breastfeed in toilets out of fear they'll be judged for the opposite. How depressing is it that no matter what you do, there's a version of social shame waiting for you?

Maybe you couldn't breastfeed. Maybe you didn't want to. Maybe formula saved your sanity. Whatever your reasons, they are yours and you do not owe anyone an explanation.

Before I had a baby, I hoped I'd be able to breastfeed, but I also knew that I might not be able to. However, when Alfie arrived, we took to it straight away. Don't get me wrong, it was painful, and we had to work really hard to keep his weight up, but I was surprised by how much I loved it. After years of having my breasts objectified and sexualised, breastfeeding gave them a new kind of purpose. For the first time, they weren't being stared at or commented on; they were feeding my baby. That felt powerful. I couldn't believe that my body had been his home for nine months and was still nourishing him now.

Learning about breastfeeding blew my mind. When a baby suckles, a small amount of their saliva is transferred back into the nipple; this so-called 'baby backwash' gives the mother's body information about the baby's health. If they're fighting an infection, her milk can adjust to provide more antibodies. The human body is magic! But I found myself feeling increasingly lonely, especially as the months rolled on. In the UK, only around 1 per cent of babies are exclusively breastfed after six months.[30] I watched mums around me return to their lives, able to leave their babies with partners or caregivers, while I stayed home, tethered to my child. Before I had a baby, I would say that I'd never be one of 'those mums' who couldn't be separated from their child, and yet here I was. It made me question if I was doing it all wrong. Friends stopped inviting me to things – they knew I wouldn't be able to come, but it still stung.

If I ever mentioned how isolated I was becoming, or how much I missed my old life and how different my new normal looked compared to others who leave the house without their babies, people would dismiss me. 'Just give him a bottle,' they said. But it wasn't that simple – I couldn't. I tried every bottle on the market (literally), but Alfie refused them all. (I've since found out he has an undiagnosed lip and tongue tie, which explains a lot in hindsight.) Breastfeeding can be beautiful and bonding and still feel suffocating. It can be empowering and exhausting all at once. And the real kicker? You're still judged for doing it, even by healthcare professionals.

Once, I was feeding Alfie at a family-friendly attraction when a member of staff asked me to move to the toilet. 'Would you eat your lunch in a toilet?' I asked. Another time I was giving Ada her first feed in hospital shortly after her birth. I was waiting to be moved to another ward, and the staff kept asking me if I wanted to cover up, warning me that other people would see me. All these tiny comments reinforce the idea that breastfeeding is something private. The idea that breastfeeding is 'intimate' or 'inappropriate' only makes sense if you view women's bodies as sexual objects first and functional bodies second. Plus, babies feed constantly, and if you had to do every feed in private, you'd never leave the house. Way to empower new mums!

Online, it was worse. In those early months, the only time I could really be on my phone was when I sat down to breastfeed, so I would chat away on my Instagram stories, seeking connection and companionship. In response, I was slut-shamed and called an attention seeker for appearing onscreen while breastfeeding. The same old tired tropes I'd heard since my teens. *Who do you think I want attention from in this scenario?* I'd think. It just confirmed what I already knew: we still struggle to see breasts as anything other than sexual.

If you're breastfeeding, or hoping to, know that you have every right to feed your baby *anywhere* in public. It's protected under the Equality Act 2010 and it's illegal for anyone to ask you to leave a public place. It doesn't matter whether it's a bus, in a hospital, in a café. Or even national television!

In fact, I breastfed on *The Jeremy Vine Show*. It was my first time back in a television studio post-lockdown. I couldn't leave Alfie, but I was scared my career would disappear if I kept turning down opportunities. I needed people to remember that I was still the same Ashley James, and not 'just a mum'. Not that society should think there's anything unworthy about being a full-time parent! Tommy took the morning off to wait with Alfie in the greenroom, and the production team reassured me that, if he got hungry or upset, he could come on set, even if we were live. Sure enough, he ended up coming out and rooting for a feed, so I fed him. By then, it felt completely normal to me – I'd been doing it for months. But, inside, I felt crushed. This was supposed to be my moment to prove I was the same old Ashley, and instead I was the mum breastfeeding live on telly.

But when I look back now, I'm really proud of that moment. I hope it helped normalise what so many mums are doing every single day – trying to balance their babies' needs with their own ambitions. I also hope it served as a reminder that breastfeeding is normal, unremarkable and unpredictable. I breastfed Alfie for twelve months and only stopped when he started biting me.

Before Ada arrived, I wasn't sure I could go through it all again. Not just the time and sacrifice, but the accusations and constant commentary around my body. Although it made me feel sad that I was made to feel shame or worry for something that others are shamed for not doing. I felt guilty even considering not breastfeeding her, but I wasn't in lockdown anymore and life was faster and busier, especially with a toddler in tow and no maternity leave. I had to trust that things would work out however they were meant to, and they did. I ended up breastfeeding her for fourteen months, but Ada was a very different baby. It was much easier to go out, work and socialise as she fed less, and she'd happily take a bottle too. She came with me to DJ at Ministry of Sound and even travelled with me to Leeds when I filmed *Steph's Packed Lunch*. I loved our little adventures together.

I'm proud of my breastfeeding journeys, but I wish they hadn't been so controversial. I hate that feeding choices are a battleground. I wish it hadn't made me feel like I constantly had to explain myself, justify myself or apologise. Sophie Ellis-Bextor once said to me, 'Just remember, no one sits around talking about how long you breastfed your kids once they're older.' And she's right. It feels like the most defining part of early motherhood while you're in it, and then, one day, it's not even something that comes up. So feed your baby however works for you, whether that's breast, bottle or both. All will have challenges, and we all deserve support, not judgement.

The same goes for sleep. Before I had kids, I used to say things like, 'Mums don't own tiredness! I'm allowed to be tired too.' And that's obviously true. I'd felt tiredness before becoming a parent. When I was pregnant, I'd say, 'I'm a DJ. I'm used to late nights, so the sleep deprivation doesn't scare me.' And that's also true. I knew what it felt like to be sleep deprived. Or, at least, I thought I did. In the first few weeks of Alfie's life, I'd say things like, 'Oh, I'm tired, but the tiredness is so worth it.' And it was. I'll never forget those magical moments, just me and my baby in the dark as the rest of the world slept.

But then, as the months passed and Alf still wasn't sleeping, I realised this wasn't DJ tired. It wasn't the same tiredness as pushing through a hangover. Life with a baby meant there were no days off. No lie-ins. It was never-ending, night after night after night. Because Alfie didn't sleep much, we ended up co-sleeping, both out of choice and sheer survival. He just slept better cuddled up next to me, which meant I also slept better. And I got it. He'd been snuggled up inside me for nine months; I was his home, why wouldn't he want to be close to me?

Unfortunately, co-sleeping is another parenting taboo that is frowned upon and critiqued – even when parents take steps to manage any risks. Even though most new breastfeeding mothers today don't plan to bedshare, studies show that 60 to 75 per cent of them end up doing so at least some of the time.[31] So, however it's judged, the two often go hand in hand.

Sleep seemed to be the only topic of conversation in every baby group I went to, and it turned out that my sleep habits with my baby were very much in the minority. Everyone was talking about sleep training and 'crying it out', and I was told I was 'creating a rod for my own back' by following my instincts. I felt like I couldn't talk to anyone, and when I did break down with exhaustion, the message was: well, you chose this.

I didn't want to 'fix' my baby. I wanted to respond to him. Because I had chosen not to sleep train, the judgement and advice to abandon my gut was relentless. And yet I stuck with it, not because I thought it was better, but because I couldn't bear to do anything else. The truth is that co-sleeping and responsive night-time parenting have been practised for centuries and are still the norm in many parts of the world. In the West, we often shame parents for following those instincts and tell them it's dangerous. Yet even in the UK, children only began to sleep in their own rooms during the late nineteenth century, when medical anxieties about disease transmission gained currency. The modern expectation for solitary sleep is rooted in Western industrialisation and ideas of independence, not in biology or emotional need.

What did give me a huge sense of comfort was knowing that Tommy's mum was also always responsive – day and night – and all her four children are very secure. On the hard days (and nights), that did give me hope. I'm not trying to say that everyone should do it the way I did it. I look back now and wonder if I struggled for too long. But I'm also really proud to know I made it through. I followed my intuition and I did it with confidence.

Sleep train or don't sleep train, but don't judge others for their choices.

What else have I been judged for? Oh, childcare! I am still to this day constantly judged for paying for childcare, but how else are we meant to work *and* look after our children? When I tried to make that impossible riddle work, I ended up feeling I was failing at both. When Alfie wouldn't take a bottle, I hired a nanny so that I could feed him between work, and I received so much negative pushback. Nannies are stigmatised, even though they can be as affordable as a nursery if you have more than one child. Plus, they are much more flexible for people who don't work traditional hours. Even now that my children are in a nursery, there is still judgement. Childcare is a necessity for working mothers, not a luxury. 'Don't give up your dreams and aspirations,' we're told, but also 'Don't bother having children if you're going to outsource looking after them.' Never be on your phone, but stay on top of friendships and relationships. Never leave your baby with anyone else, but don't be one of *those* mums who makes her whole world about her kids. We're meant to work like we don't have kids and bring up children like we don't work. It's just one trap after another.

People have made barbed comments about me 'letting other people raise my children', feedback that has never been directed to Tommy. He isn't asked who's looking after the kids while he works. He's not judged for going back to the office. No one accuses him of bad habits or critiques him on how his kids are fed or sleeping. He's free to just get on with it – and celebrated for changing a single nappy. *So* 'hands on'!

Time has moved on from the traditional gendered roles of the 1950s, but the expectations are still stuck there. We're left navigating an impossible maze of contradictions, paradoxes and internalised guilt, while being judged for every turn we take.

41.
I'm a Mum's Mum

There is no single right way to do motherhood. We're all building our own puzzles with a completely different set of pieces, and just when we think we've worked it out, life throws in a new shape we didn't expect. I could tell you how I put my puzzle together, but it wouldn't help you because you will be building a totally different one.

But what I can do is try to give you the confidence to build your version. To encourage you when you're finding it hard to connect it all together and cheer you on when you find that vital corner piece. And I hope you would help me back. Our puzzles all look different depending on our circumstances, our preferences, our support networks, and our own strengths and weaknesses, but we all share a common truth: we're trying to be good parents in a system that doesn't support us and judges us no matter what we do.

So that's why I now say: I'm a mum's mum. I won't judge you, because I know you are doing what you think is right. I will listen to you when you tell me your struggles. No matter how you parent, I trust that you know what's best for your child. I won't give unsolicited advice, but, if you ask, I'll offer it with love. I want you to trust your gut, not the guilt.

My sister and I had our first babies four months apart. Her

experience was completely different to mine. She's a stay-at-home mum and an army wife with no nearby family support and little disposable income to outsource help. I work full-time and rely on childcare in order to do so. I breastfed, while my sister couldn't, despite desperately trying. She tormented herself with the pump and guilt until she realised formula was what worked for her baby – and her sanity. Watching her suffer under the pressure of a narrative that says you're not trying hard enough if you don't breastfeed broke my heart. Just because I breastfed and had my own set of challenges, it didn't mean I couldn't be there for her too. She sleep trained because she was at breaking point with the nights – and I totally supported her choice.

My sister and made many different choices with our babies, but we both had challenges, and we both needed support. And we both faced judgement no matter what we did – me for breastfeeding, her for bottle-feeding. Me for co-sleeping, her for sleep training. But we never judged each other, because we understood that our babies, our lives, our circumstances, were different. Her baby needed one thing. Mine needed another. She needed rest to function. I needed reassurance that my baby was okay sleeping beside me. We both made our choices out of love.

There's no gold medal for how you get through the nights or days of early motherhood, only the hope that you can. Both of our babies are now happy toddlers in loving homes. We tried to uplift each other and be there night and day through our own unique realities. Isn't that what every new parent deserves?

So, no, I don't care how you feed your baby. Or how you get them to sleep. Or whether you go back to work or stay home. I care that you feel supported. That you feel seen. That you have choices and aren't made to feel ashamed of them.

I'm a mum's mum.

Every time we battle each other, we put our frustration and energy in the wrong place. The real problem is the patriarchal systems that are failing us and preventing us from thriving. We have to fight the system, not each other.

Rather than wasting time debating how we nourish our children, we should be fighting to ensure that every woman who wants to breastfeed has access to the help, time and support to do so, and every woman who bottle feeds feels safe to do so in every space.

Rather than judging each other's childcare choices we should be demanding an affordable system that works for everyone. Having two children at nursery full-time in London costs us £4,000 a month, and fees have risen 7 per cent in the last year. That is a privilege most people can't afford, and while I feel immensely fortunate that we can pay that, I also feel angry that we have to just so we can do our jobs.

It's not really any surprise that, in the UK, 74,000 women a year can't afford to return to work due to the cost of childcare and lack of flexibility. That means 74,000 individuals who want to work are unable to do so. That's 74,000 women financially dependent on partners. That's 74,000 women who are giving up holiday pay, sickness protections and future pension contributions. That's 74,000 women who are forced into traditional gender roles they may not have chosen. Who risk being accused of 'taking half' if they ever want to leave.

In countries like Norway and Germany, generous paid leave, subsidised childcare and flexible work policies mean women aren't forced to choose between their careers and their children. Imagine what we could do if we came together to demand a better system so that people who choose to go back to work are able to, and people who choose to stay at home can too?

Choice is the whole point of feminism. I often think about how much I would hate to be a stay-at-home mum. I'm so grateful to all the women who came before me who fought for my right to be able to pursue my career dreams. But I also acknowledge that it might be your dream. I love that for you, and I want you to be able to follow your aspirations. I also want housewives and stay-at-home mums to have the recognition – and respect – they deserve in society. How we've let anyone dare tell us that it is 'not working' is beyond me. It's societal gaslighting of the highest degree! Since becoming a mum, going to work feels like a break, not the other way around. Commuting on the tube and listening to my own music with no one shouting for my attention feels like a spa break in comparison.

Even though Tommy and I can afford childcare, we still spend the week juggling the logistics of pick-ups, drop-offs, inset days and school picnics. Because in the end we're all trying to fill in the cracks of a system that was never designed to support working women. It's a reminder that motherhood is just another space where women are judged and stretched impossibly thin by patriarchal systems that shrink rather than empower us. Once I realised that I couldn't win, I found I was liberated. I saw that I might as well do it all my own way, guilt-free. So, here's to trusting our instincts and inspiring other mums to follow theirs, judgement-free.

I want us to stop defending our decisions and start defending each other. We need to stop being each other's critics and start being each other's lifelines. We need to recognise that no matter what we choose, all paths come with challenges. And the most important thing is to protect our right to *choose*. We're not each other's enemies and the more we come together, the more impossible it becomes for the system to ignore us.

HYSTERICAL
hɪˈstɛr.ɪ.kəl
adjective

a term historically used to label women as irrational, overly emotional or mentally unstable, often as a way to dismiss or undermine them. Its roots lie in the Greek word *hystera*. They believed that a 'wandering womb' was the cause of many medical issues in women. But it was the Victorians who tied female 'hysteria' to madness and translated it into a medical diagnosis used to pathologise normal female emotions or behaviour. Women who showed anger, grief, sexuality or ambition could be deemed 'hysterical' and sometimes even institutionalised.

Male equivalent: There is no true male equivalent. Men who express intense emotion are more likely to be called *passionate*, *driven* or *stressed*. Their feelings are seen as situational; women's are seen as innate flaws. *Hysterical* is a word that has long been used to discredit women's pain or protest, reducing them to caricatures of instability. Its legacy lingers in how women are still told to 'calm down' or accused of 'overreacting', especially when challenging authority or injustice.

42.
Ruining Your Body

Historically, a woman's value and worth was tied to her fertility, and even now we see how much power structures and labels push women into having babies. We are warned against becoming a 'crazy cat lady', told we'll regret not having children, and asked who will look after us when we're older. And yet, despite being told that motherhood is the most important thing we can do, there is so much shame and misogynistic social commentary surrounding pregnant and postnatal bodies.

When I first discovered I was pregnant, I took photos of my body from all angles so I could remember what it looked like before it was 'ruined forever'. I'd look at my reflection and wonder how pregnancy would change me. Would my body be unrecognisable? Would I ever feel like myself again? So many of us experience these fears because they stem from a culture that makes women believe their looks define their worth and convinces us our value diminishes if we don't 'snap back' to our pre-baby bodies within weeks of giving birth.

I was also anxious about the whole vaginal-tightness situation. I'm cringing as I write this, because honestly! But, hey, that was what I worried about. I've since learned that as your vagina is an actual muscle, any changes in tone or elasticity are often temporary. This idea that vaginas are permanently 'loose' after childbirth is exaggerated and rooted in misinformation and misogyny. I was aware of 'tight vaginas' being a topic of conversation between boys and then men ever since high school. The cultural obsession comes from the long history of centring male pleasure. Tightness is perceived as more pleasurable for men and therefore more desirable. The myth is tangled up in toxic ideas about virginity, with 'tight' made synonymous with pure, clean and untouched. GROSS. It's also worth mentioning that when a woman is aroused, her vagina naturally lubricates and expands. So, if she's tight, it could actually suggest she might not be that into it. It's called a clitoris, mate, google it!

During pregnancy, a body does miraculous things: it grows an entirely new organ (the placenta), expands to accommodate a baby, and develops the ability to sustain another human being. After birth, it heals itself, adjusts to new hormonal realities, and, for many women, even produces milk to nourish their baby. Every stretch mark, scar or change is a testament to this incredible journey. But, sure, we've 'ruined' our bodies.

When you really think about that phrase, it reveals how society values women's bodies primarily for their appearance over their strength, capability and function. It completely ignores the incredible ways our bodies adapt, grow and work tirelessly to create and nurture life through pregnancy, childbirth and beyond. The idea that we destroy our figures is so toxic, and I think it reflects some of the negative societal attitudes we hold towards mothers – as if, once we've fulfilled our purpose to procreate, we're somehow 'spoiled'. Once we have a baby, we are no longer desirable to men and are given a new set of expectations to adhere to. We're no longer allowed to wear certain clothes, and we must carry ourselves in a way that is 'appropriate' for a mother. It doesn't matter that nearly all of us become mothers by having sex; once we have procreated, we are no longer allowed to express our sexuality. 'She's a mother now,' they will say. Although, interestingly, the same moral expectations are never placed on dads.

For as long as we continue to use these phrases, each generation keeps adopting these attitudes.

Yet despite all the concerns about ruining our bodies, we are told to enjoy our pregnancies. For my part, I absolutely loved my first pregnancy. I mean, the boob pain wasn't ideal in the first trimester, and I had to sleep in sports bras, but apart from that, it was great. I was tired, but given we were in lockdown, and I had no other children, I had the luxury of napping whenever I wanted. That year gave us a beautiful summer, so I got lots of sunshine and sleep.

As I entered my second trimester, I felt euphoric. I've never felt so at one with Mother Nature. You know when Snow White is surrounded by animals? That's how I felt. While I wasn't exactly ensconced in a forest – I'm not sure being surrounded by foxes and rats in a city gives quite the same vibe – I definitely felt connected to something beyond my body. I had so much energy, I felt really body confident as my little bump started to show, and I just felt blessed. Even my cravings were healthy: I'd demolish cherry tomatoes like there was no tomorrow.

One of my neighbours was a personal trainer who, like the rest of us, was unable to work. His balcony looked onto mine, and he would guide me through gentle exercises, which I kept up throughout my pregnancy, determined to remain fit and strong so I could have a 'good birth and quick recovery'. That's what I was told would happen, so that's what I expected.

Then came the third trimester and everything shifted. I developed something called Pelvic Girdle Pain (PGP), a type of agony that occurs in the joints and ligaments of the pelvis. It's especially common during pregnancy, thanks to a combination of hormonal changes, such as the increased concentration of relaxin released to loosen ligaments in preparation for childbirth, as well as postural changes as your centre of gravity realigns. Weight gain, pressure on the pelvis, muscle imbalances, and a weak core or pelvic floor can also all contribute to it. For me, it was excruciating. Everything became challenging, from turning over in bed, getting up, walking, climbing stairs – even standing on one leg. I was given a pelvic brace and had to carry a carrier bag around. Pelvic girdle pain tip: always carry a plastic bag so you can sit on it and spin yourself out of a car like a rotisserie chicken. All that exercise stopped, and suddenly I felt restricted within my body.

There are so many things we don't account for in pregnancy, so many common issues for which there is close to zero cultural understanding. We all hear about morning sickness, but the minute you experience it, you learn the joke is in the name. How about we call it all-day-and-all-night sickness? Or never-ending sickness? Lots of women also experience hyperemesis gravidarum, which is extreme sickness during pregnancy, something that is finally getting a little more public recognition because the Princess of Wales experienced it. It can lead to debilitating physical and mental health decline for so many women. The anxiety that can come with pregnancy, especially for women who've experienced baby loss, ectopic pregnancies or terminations for medical reasons, can be severe. Some women become deeply depressed. Hormonal shifts can cause acne breakouts, wild water retention or hugely swollen feet, and many of us experience painful cramps or Braxton Hicks contractions for long stretches.

So, when women are told to 'enjoy their pregnancy' or

be grateful to be pregnant, it can feel like they're being gaslit. You wouldn't wish HG on your worst enemy. For some, pregnancy is just not an enjoyable experience, and we need to be able to hold space and compassion for each other without judgement or guilt. Sure, some women enjoy their pregnancy, like I did at first. But others endure it with gritted teeth. We can be grateful to be creating a longed-for baby and still be counting down the days until it's over. There should be no guilt or remorse because pregnancies are incomparable.

My third trimester marked the beginning of my realisation that motherhood isn't something you can control or plan, no matter how much you might want to. Our bodies, our births, our babies – they can all have totally different ideas to the visions we have for ourselves.

Towards the end of my pregnancy, I wasn't glowing. I wasn't floating around in a linen dress with flowers in my hair, feeling connected to the universe. I was in pain. I was fed up. I just wanted this baby out. Maybe nature makes us feel like that so we actually look forward to the birth.

My hospital bags were packed, and I was ready to say goodbye to my pregnancy body. But nothing could have quite prepared me for what came next. I was about to learn about the systemic medical neglect and poor maternity care that impacts so many of us up and down the country.

43.
Negative Birth Stories

'You only ever hear negative birth stories' is one of the biggest trigger phrases for me. And I say this as someone who definitely said that while I was pregnant the first time around. Back then, I felt that the fear mongering and catastrophising were endemic in the media and online, and I was almost annoyed with other mothers for their bleak portrayal of birth, so deeply ingrained were my misogynistic attitudes. I was happier to dismiss and blame women for their poor mindset than show compassion for their experience or question why so many seemed to be so mentally scarred by their births.

I now know these 'negative birth stories' are actually individual people's traumatic experiences. If someone has a car accident, we'd never tell them that people have been getting into cars for years without complaining. We wouldn't minimise their pain or trauma by telling them they should be grateful they're alive. We wouldn't sneer when they said they needed pain relief, nor would we compare their experience to someone else who got through it without medication. In fact, if someone told me they'd had any other operation or procedure without pain relief, I would wonder what was wrong with them. Is this masochism? And yet, mums are praised for giving birth as if we're in the Stone Age when medicine didn't exist. It's *absolutely bizarre* when you break it down.

While I was pregnant, I took hypnobirthing classes and very much adopted its techniques as my blueprint for birth. For anyone unfamiliar, hypnobirthing is a childbirth preparation method that teaches relaxation, visualisation and breathing exercises to promote a calmer and more comfortable birth. The idea is that fear and tension make labour harder and more painful. This is factually correct – oxytocin drives uterine contractions that dilate the cervix and move the baby down the birth canal, and adrenaline and stress can hinder oxytocin. I *loved* hypnobirthing in theory. While it doesn't promise a completely pain-free birth, it does focus on making it feel more empowering and manageable rather than frightening. At the time, it gave me so much confidence going into labour. Yet, now, it leaves a sour taste in my mouth.

The techniques are undeniably helpful, and many women apply them to other areas of their life well after birth. But the logic that drives it seems to contribute to the idea that if your birth ends up going wrong, somehow you are to blame. If only you'd stayed calm. If only you'd breathed better. I often sit and squirm as people tell me they had a positive birth *because* they did hypnobirthing. While I always celebrate positive birth experiences, a low-drama birth isn't only down to mindset, breath patterns and high levels of oxytocin. There are so many other variable factors that are totally out of your control.

Before I got pregnant, I'd run two marathons, both with very little training. For one of them, I'd got off a plane the day before after a week partying at Coachella. Jetlag and party lag is not ideal marathon prep. But I knew how to push my body and my mind through pain. I knew I had grit. Thanks to the birthing courses, I knew how important it was to advocate for myself. I knew my options around drugs and how birth was supposed to unfold. I was excited. Excited to meet the love of my life I'd been carrying. Excited to not have PGP. Honestly, I was even excited to go through birth and see what the mystery was about. Up until then, I'd only ever seen the words 'mother and baby doing well'. What does 'well' even mean? How can she be doing well when she just pushed a baby out of her vagina? Well! I was about to find out that 'well' is a very loose term post-birth, basically meaning . . . not in a coma or dead.

My due date was 3 January. I really hoped he'd be born on the 31 December or 1 January, firstly as that was our anniversary, and secondly because I thought people would always be up for celebrating his birthday. Unlike my sister who is mid-January and is constantly told everyone's either broke or doing Dry Jan. But babies don't care about your plans, they do what they want.

No one prepares you for the feeling of being overdue. Waking up every day wondering, 'Will it be today?' Going to bed wondering, 'Will it be tonight?' Feeling more uncomfortable with every passing twenty-four hours. Getting endless 'any news?' messages from everyone in your phonebook. I tried everything to get that baby out. All the old wives' tales! Reflexology, spicy food, dates, raspberry leaf tea, orgasms (ironically the only time society ever encourages female pleasure). I got angry at Tommy when he said he couldn't physically have sex with me. 'I can see the baby right there,' he said. 'I honestly don't think I could even if I wanted to.'

'DO YOU WANT ME TO STAY PREGNANT FOR EVER? PLEASE DO YOUR BIT!'

My contractions started around 7 p.m. on 8 January. Knowing Alf now, it makes sense; he does things in his own time. It was a few days into the third national lockdown, which definitely didn't help my stress levels. People had been allowed to play golf and sit outdoors in pubs, but we didn't know if partners were allowed with us during childbirth.

We were watching *Once Upon a Time in Hollywood* when I felt something happening. *Finally!* I started to track my contractions on the app as I'd been taught, and text my midwife. I decided to get some sleep, knowing it might be my last chance for a few days – or eighteen years – then I woke up again at 2 a.m. as the contractions ramped up. We jumped in a taxi to take the ten-minute journey to the hospital and that's when it started to really hurt. It wasn't the pain of the contractions themselves, although of course they weren't a walk in the park. But they were what I'd expected: cyclical surges of pain with peaks. The issue was a different pain entirely . . . a constant and steady pain that never went away.

When we arrived, Tommy was asked to wait outside. Even to this day, I still feel so angry about the fact that so many of us had to give birth without partners, especially given the vast majority of them were living with us. Mothers were let down during the pandemic, but I suppose I shouldn't have been surprised!

I was having regular contractions and explained I was in *constant* pain. Not grit-your-teeth pain. More bite-your-fist-so-you-don't-scream pain. My course had taught me that physical checks were optional, however I was told that, due to pandemic rules, if I wanted Tommy in the room with me, they'd need to physically check how dilated I was. They also said they needed to see how far along I was to know what pain relief options were available to me. I agreed as, in theory, I had no issue with this cervix check, but the moment they began, I thought I was going to pass out. The pain was unexpectedly *unbearable*. I asked them to stop twice, but they told me in no uncertain terms that they needed to continue. It still haunts me that I went through that without even a paracetamol. The only consolation was that Tommy was finally allowed in.

Hours passed and I was slowly becoming convinced that I was going to die. I *begged*, *pleaded*, *wailed* for pain relief, but the promise of an epidural never came. When I desperately asked for a C-section, I was told it was off the table. Eventually, after hours and hours of grovelling, I was given pethidine. It didn't take the pain away, but at least it made me drowsy. The moment that broke me was when the midwife team told me they were going to go home for a nap and would be back before the birth. It had already been *hours*. Where did they live? How long were they napping for? How much longer was I going to be left in this pain? I DON'T CARE WHAT I SAID ON THE BIRTH PLAN, GET THIS BABY OUT OF ME. I'd been led to believe I had choices. We'd packed fairy lights. WTF WAS THIS?! And why on earth had I packed fairy lights?

Eventually, after several more hours, it was time to go, and I pushed harder than I've ever pushed myself in my whole life. I'm pretty sure I didn't even wait for the contractions. Tommy still remembers the sound of my vagina tearing. The pushing pain was what I'd imagined, hard but manageable. Shortly after 1 p.m. on 9 January, my beautiful baby boy Alfie Rivers took his first breath. He came out blue. But thank goodness he was here, and he was okay. I didn't get that 'love at first sight' moment; instead I just felt relief that he was here, and it was over. When I looked at him, I remember just thinking how purple he was rather than the magical rush of bonding I'd been promised.

That day is still one of the most traumatic experiences of my life, although I didn't realise it at the time. Back then, I was just thankful that we had both made it through. That he was here. Alive. That I wasn't in pain anymore.

The real test didn't come for me until much later. I want to say clearly that while I see my birth as traumatic, I don't see it as negative. Not because I did anything wrong. Not because I didn't advocate for myself or know my options or breathe properly. I wasn't scared about childbirth, I was fit and mentally strong. I wasn't seeking any kind of badge of honour. But this experience changed me. It made me lose trust in our medical care. It poisoned my journey into motherhood through its sheer barbarism. I was dismissed, infantilised and stripped of any kind of agency. Every ounce of the confidence that I had in my body was torn away. I now don't feel stories like this are negative. I feel they are spoken to try to hold the system accountable for the way it fails and degrades women.

I am not the first, and I won't be the last, to have a difficult birth experience. Although, of course, so many have endured far worse, with less happy outcomes than mine. Black women are three times more likely to die in pregnancy and childbirth,[32] twice as likely to experience a stillbirth,[33] and 43 per cent more likely to experience a miscarriage.[34]

The problem is that birth isn't something you can just go back and do again. Months later, when I did my birth debrief (something we can all request to do for free after a birth, along with requesting our birth notes through the NHS), I asked why I was denied pain relief. I was fully prepared for a practical reason, such as staffing issues, or maybe that there were no anaesthetists to carry out the epidural. It *was* during a pandemic, after all. Those answers wouldn't have made it right, but they might have given me some sense of acceptance, although I'd still have preferred to have been given a straight-up answer during the birth.

But no. The very kind lady on the call told me that, in fact, the notes said I wasn't given pain relief because I was – and

I quote – 'coping fine'. I burst out crying. How could they possibly have said that? I'd hoped for closure, but that sentence made me feel even worse. How could they possibly have written that? How could they have interpreted my absolute desperation – *my begging, pleading, wailing* – as being 'fine'? I even asked Tommy if there was any doubt in his mind that I was coping? I couldn't have been clearer: I was in pain. And yet they chose to ignore me and then rewrote history with intentional deception. Let me say once again for the record, I was a long way from 'fine'.

Whether we have a high or a low pain threshold shouldn't really matter. Pain is deeply personal and entirely subjective – no one else can truly know how it feels in your body. In labour, this becomes especially important, because what looks manageable from the outside might feel overwhelming on the inside. Too often, women's requests for pain relief are brushed aside because we've been conditioned to suck it up and not wail like banshees. Your pain is valid because you feel it – not because someone in a white coat deems it serious enough. If you communicate it clearly, you deserve in every context for your voice to be heard. Or at the very least for it to be recorded.

Of course, in any birth setting, midwives and doctors have a responsibility to weigh up pain relief options and the well-being of the baby. But that should never come at the cost of dismissing the birthing person. You deserve to be spoken to like an adult – with respect, clear explanations and compassion. If something you've asked for isn't immediately possible, you should be told why and given support to manage in the meantime. Birth is not just about getting the baby out safely; it's also about how *you* are treated and how *you* feel in that room. Being heard shouldn't be a bonus; it's a basic right.

44.
The Gender Pain Gap

During my birth debrief, I was told about the Ockenden Report – a major independent review into maternity care failings at the Shrewsbury and Telford Hospital NHS Trust, led by midwife Donna Ockenden. The final report, published in March 2022, three months before my birth debrief, exposed decades of serious and repeated failures in maternity care, leading to the avoidable deaths and harm of mothers and babies. Countless women and children had been affected because they weren't listened to, because concerns were brushed aside, and because the system prioritised image over safety.

In several cases, women were denied pain relief when they had asked clearly and firmly for it. Some were spoken to dismissively or even cruelly. The report concluded that at least 201 babies and nine mothers may have survived if better care had been provided. She also reassured me that things were changing because the report had served as a powerful wake-up call across the UK. It exposed how dangerous things become when women aren't heard, when safety is sacrificed for ideology, and when systems protect medical staff at the expense of their patients. It also highlighted how essential it is to engage with women, provide truly informed consent, and create maternity care that is both safe *and* respectful.

It was the first time I felt like what had happened to me wasn't just 'one of those things'. It was part of a broader pattern, and maybe, *slowly*, that story was starting to shift. The health provider on the call also told me she was on the board for the vaginal mesh scandal, one of the most significant women's health crises in the UK in recent history, and one you may not even have heard of. It involved thousands of women being injured by transvaginal mesh implants, used to treat pelvic organ dysfunction or stress urinary incontinence, both often a result of childbirth (more on that shortly).

These mesh devices, made of synthetic material, were supposed to act as internal support structures. But, instead, many women experienced devastating complications. What made the scandal even worse was how women were treated when they spoke up. Many reported being dismissed, gaslit or belittled by doctors. Some were told the pain was 'in their head', that they were 'overreacting', or that they simply had to 'put up with it' because they were getting older or had children. These sexist, minimising comments implied that women's suffering was either exaggerated or just a normal part of being female – rather than a sign of serious medical harm. One woman recalled being told, 'You're a woman – what do you expect?' while others were labelled 'hysterical' for insisting something was wrong.

I loathe the word 'hysterical', because it's been weaponised against us, generation after generation. It comes from the word 'hystera', which is Greek for uterus. For centuries, 'female hysteria' was considered a legitimate medical diagnosis. As far back as 1900 BC, ancient texts claimed a woman's uterus could roam around her body causing all sorts of mischief, from anxiety to madness. Treatments focused on luring it back to its 'rightful place'. But 'hysteria' really took off in the nineteenth century – conveniently, around the same time the women's rights movement was gathering momentum. The first women's rights convention was held in the US in 1850; by 1859, physicians (almost exclusively men, and often without formal training) were claiming that *one in four women* suffered from hysteria.

What better way to silence a woman demanding equality than to declare her irrational?

Obviously, women were far too emotional to be trusted with money, jobs, degrees or votes. We were biologically unstable. That was the line – and society swallowed it.

The problem was, in those days, a married woman could be committed to an asylum without any trial or evidence. If her husband said she was insane, that was enough. Many women were locked up simply for disagreeing with their husbands, wanting a divorce or showing signs of distress or pain – often because they were experiencing actual abuse. But under the law, they weren't victims. They were mad, *hysterical* in fact.

You could be diagnosed with hysteria for almost anything: being anxious or irritable, having too much of a libido or not enough, being too loud, too opinionated, too smart, too tired, reading too much, dressing sloppily, studying anything intellectual, having your period, not having your period, being pregnant, breastfeeding, menopausal or infertile. Basically, being a woman.

Victorian doctors genuinely believed that menstruation could make you insane. Girls were given cold baths and told to avoid meat in an effort to delay puberty. And if you were a Black woman, simply wanting freedom from slavery could be seen as a sign of insanity, because slavery was supposedly 'good for you'. Because hysteria was thought to originate in the womb, the treatments focused on women's sexual organs.

Some were horrifying: ice water injected into vaginas, leeches attached to labia and clitorises, caustic chemicals applied to genitals. Vaginal exams became standard, and chloroform was used to 'quiet' outspoken women.

The most infamous treatment was clitoridectomy. In the 1860s, Dr Isaac Baker Brown, a senior London surgeon, wrote an entire book advocating for cutting off women's clitorises to 'cure' hysteria. He performed the procedure on countless women and girls. Why? Because it made them more obedient – in and out of the bedroom. He even suggested it as an alternative to divorce. The last recorded case of clitoridectomy for 'emotional issues' was performed in the 1940s on a *five-year-old girl*. Another common 'cure' was removing a woman's ovaries – hence the term hysterectomy. A woman was considered healed when she became quiet, submissive, modest and well-dressed.

In other words, broken.

Depressingly, this isn't just some grim nineteenth-century footnote. Hysteria remained a formal psychiatric diagnosis in the DSM – the official manual of mental disorders – until 1980.

My experience was a reminder and valuable lesson that our pain is still so often dismissed. We are still so often told we are 'coping fine' or that we are being 'crazy' when, to anyone with eyes, we are clearly not. Whether it's menopause, childbirth, endometriosis, IBS, getting the coil fitted or any of the other myriad of health issues that you may suffer from, don't let anyone tell you it's 'in your head'.

It is a scandal how so many women are abandoned after childbirth in this country. We are left traumatised (and not just by the birth, but by the feeling of total and utter powerlessness), having been treated as failures, or weaklings who can't make the grade in the ultimate test of womanhood. I can't imagine a more aggressive assault on a woman's confidence. With no care, no frank advice, not even basic acknowledgement of the injuries we might have suffered, we are sent home and thrown in at the deep end of the most important, stressful and exhausting job we will ever do. And because we are so vulnerable, because our recovery and any post-birth damage is so shrouded in shame, we don't fight back.

We will never improve things if we continue to focus on women's failures rather than the governments who are stripping our public health services and destroying our NHS. Women should never be silent, because the louder our voices and the more we demand systemic changes, the better things will become.

45.
A 'Positive Birth Story'

I didn't want to have a caesarean birth the first time around. I'm not entirely sure why, but I think I'd absorbed a lot of the messaging that C-sections weren't 'real' births. That they were for women who were *too posh to push* or had low pain thresholds. Two years and two months after Alfie, I chose to have a caesarean and it finally allowed me to experience the beauty of a positive birth.

I say I 'chose' a C-section, and that's partly true. But I was also medically advised not to give birth vaginally due to the injuries which I'd sustained (more on this to come) in my first delivery. You didn't need to ask me twice. People are often judgemental of C-sections because of deeply rooted beliefs about childbirth shaped by outdated gender roles and romanticised ideas of motherhood. For centuries, women were praised for labouring in silence and seen as more virtuous if they gave birth naturally, without complaint or intervention. The idea that childbirth pain is 'deserved female punishment' stems from religion, especially Christianity and Judaism (hello, Eve and the apple!), and enduring it became a kind of moral currency. That legacy still lingers. The 'ideal' birth is often imagined as vaginal, unmedicated and mystical; something sacred that connects mother and baby through instinct alone. Anything medicalised can be seen as a failure to live up to that ideal. C-sections, especially planned ones, are perceived by some as taking a shortcut. As if birth is a test of endurance or proof of the validity of our womanhood. This mindset turns childbirth into a competition, where strength is measured by how much pain you can take. I can tell you that, at the end of any birth, there are no prizes. We don't get medals or certificates, and whichever way you give birth, there are pros, cons and risks. C-sections are *major* abdominal surgeries, and they require a strength and bravery all of their own. The recovery can be brutal and certainly not the 'get out of jail free' card they are often painted to be.

There's also a cultural discomfort with medicalised birth. Some people see interventions as failures, as if having a C-section means your body didn't work the way it was supposed to. It's so bizarre to me that we accept medical intervention in every other area of life. When my dad had a hip replacement, no one told him to try it 'naturally', with no pain relief. No one asked him to trust his body and stay out of hospital. And yet we do that to women. Constantly.

That judgement doesn't just shape women's choices; it can cost lives. Before the Ockenden Report, some maternity wards reportedly delayed or denied necessary C-sections due to pressure to cut costs or preserve their 'natural birth' statistics. Women died. Babies died. And yet those of us who choose C-sections are made to feel ashamed. I followed my gut. I rejected lazy stereotypes and I'm so glad I did.

Making the decision to have a planned C-section gave me a blank canvas to feel excited about birth again. So, judgement about caesareans really doesn't bother me because mine allowed me to reclaim something that had been taken from me the first time: agency. That's what turned my second birth into a healing one.

I was scared of being left in pain again. So, this time, I decided to invest in private healthcare, which is obviously an incredible privilege and not something I took lightly. My doctor was incredible. She was with me from my twenty-week scan through to my birth, so I got to know her, and – more importantly – *she* got to know *me*. She knew all my trauma and worries and was able to reassure me. This is what *everyone* deserves, and it makes me so incredibly angry that we have not been able to create a system of universal care that comes even close. One of the other major factors of my choice to go private was the visiting hours system that still exists in most state hospital maternity wards. I was terrified that Tommy would be sent home almost immediately after I'd given birth. I didn't want to be left alone, especially if I had another traumatic experience. The idea that partners can be asked to leave almost immediately and not allowed back until visiting hours start again also reinforces the narrative that a baby is a mother's responsibility to look after, even after major surgery.

As the days drew closer, I couldn't wait to meet my little girl. I was excited to the point where Tommy had to keep reminding me that we weren't going away on a spa weekend. 'You *do* know you're going to give birth, right?' he said. The best part about knowing the date was being able to arrange childcare! We even booked a date at a hotel opposite the hospital the night before. This time around there were no guessing games, no old wives' tales, and no 'any news?' texts. Just peace.

On the morning of her birth, at exactly thirty-nine weeks, we walked across the road to meet our daughter. I'd made it to the date without a hint of a contraction. I was gowned up, had my catheter inserted, met the surgical team, and then lay down on the table . . . and burst into tears. Not out of fear, or sadness, but because it was *calm*. It was peaceful. I couldn't believe *this* was how it could be. I couldn't believe the moment was here.

I'd prepared a birth playlist full of soft, emotional songs. I'll never forget the moment George Ezra's 'Hold My Girl' came on and Tommy welled up. We even got to choose the song that would play as she was lifted out of my body – 'London's Song' by Matt Hartke: '*Oh my little daughter, you're the meaning of grace. I love you.*' If I could describe the feeling of having a C-section, I'd say it's like someone rummaging inside a shopping bag. But that shopping bag is your tummy. Slightly uncomfortable, but not painful. I breathed deeply, got lost in the music, and imagined my daughter.

Now, when I say I had a positive birth experience, I don't mean that everything went entirely smoothly, because it didn't. But the difference this time was communication. I was told *exactly* what was happening, in real time, adult to adult. The anaesthetist stayed by my ear and explained everything. My baby was stuck underneath my placenta. I'd known I had an anterior placenta, but they hadn't realised how low it was. If I'd tried to give birth vaginally, she would have had no way to come out. My doctor couldn't reach her, and I was losing more blood than expected. They had to use forceps to get her out and she arrived with a small cut on her face, which has thankfully healed without leaving a mark. My placenta was damaged, and they couldn't place her on my chest immediately, but I heard her crying, and I knew she was okay.

The moment she was placed on my bare chest for that skin-to-skin connection, she stopped crying. It was like she recognised my body as her home. In that instant, I felt the rush of earth-shattering, indescribable love that so many people talk about. Being stitched up was uncomfortable, but none of it mattered. She was here. She was safe. My little girl: Ada Isabella Blue.

That afternoon, Alfie came with Tommy's parents to visit us in the hospital, and later on, my friends came in and we drank champagne together until the nurse came to tell me off because I was on morphine. It was one of the best days of my life. For three days I was looked after, properly looked after, before I headed home, to begin life as a family of four.

My birthing experiences were like night and day and that is just a travesty. We shouldn't have to pay through the roof to be respected, supported and cared for. Every woman deserves to feel this safe. Every birth story deserves to be one of dignity, not survival. For me, a C-section wasn't failure, it was a chance to rewrite my story on my own terms. I look at my scar with gratitude for the positive story it tells and refuse to see it as a flaw.

46.
Baby Weight and Bouncing Back

At first, postpartum recovery seemed relatively straightforward after my first birth. I had stitches from a tear, so I was terrified of hurting myself, and equally terrified about doing that first dreaded poo. But everything felt like it was going to be all right. My understanding was that healing took about six weeks, over a period known as the 'Fourth Trimester'. Provided you were fit and healthy, you would recover well as long as you rested enough. I really did think it was that simple. And maybe for some people it is.

The only thing we ever seem to hear or read about postpartum recovery is whether or not women 'bounce back'. Bouncing or snapping back is the idea that we should return to our pre-pregnancy body, appearance and lifestyle acceptably soon after giving birth. We must defy biology and appear as if we didn't house a giant watermelon *inside* us, in among all of our internal organs. Any pounds gained in the process must be shifted sharpish. If not, we will become undesirable and find ourselves relegated to the 'she's let herself go' pile. 'Her *poor* husband,' they'll say. 'She really did let herself go after the baby, didn't she? It's always such a shame when a mum prioritises her child over her relationship!'

This narrative suggests the most impressive kind of postpartum recovery is one where there are no visible signs of the enormous physical and emotional transformation a woman has just undergone. *Delete!* The expectation is that we will sacrifice our bodies and emotions to bear children, no matter what the complication, and then mend ourselves quickly and silently, without boring anyone with unsavoury tales of struggle and negativity. On that journey, we will, we are told, regain our former confidence.

Postpartum bodies shouldn't be seen as something to be fixed or hidden. A woman who has just grown and birthed an entire human, who is likely not sleeping and possibly feeding her newborn from her own body, should never feel any pressure to try on her old jeans. Why don't we celebrate stretch marks, soft bellies, tired eyes and milk-stained tops? Why don't we worship the beauty of reality? Why aren't new mothers treated like Greek goddesses – being carried on beds while they are fed grapes and praised simply for existing? Why aren't people whispering *she made a person* with the same reverence usually reserved for miracles? Why are there not statues dedicated to the postpartum mother? How is it not desirable to embody bringing life into this world? Especially in a world that claims 'dad bods' are in fashion.

We live in a society which places so much value on thinness and shrinking ourselves that we're not even exempt from its pressures after producing a whole human being! The postpartum body, with its softness, scars, stretch marks and exposure is perceived as big, ugly, damaged and undesirable. One of my least favourite terms in the world is 'baby weight'. Referring to the weight we gain during pregnancy, while it may sound like a neutral phrase on the surface, it's often loaded with judgement, fatphobia and societal pressure. Instead of celebrating the purpose and function of that weight – growing a whole human, supporting a placenta, plus the amniotic fluid and fat reserves for breastfeeding – we view this fat as something to be ashamed of and use it as a measure for how disciplined, healthy or attractive a woman is after pregnancy.

Instead of honouring our bountiful bodies for what they have just done, we are instead scrutinised on a pretty granular level for how effectively (and quickly) we can return to a form society accepts. We have celebrity magazines and tabloid newspapers highlighting famous women's postpartum bodies. Then there's the targeted social media ads of new mothers looking slim, stylish and 'recovered' just weeks, or even days, after giving birth. I was bombarded with weight loss ads on Instagram almost immediately after leaving hospital. Cheers, Zuckerberg!

Sadly, it's not just the media that focuses on postnatal bodies; other people do too. I've had friends who lost a lot of weight naturally after giving birth. Maybe it was down to genetics, maybe it was stress, maybe it was something more complicated. Whatever the reason, they were made to feel ashamed, as if their weight loss made them complicit in creating the tangled standards for postnatal women. They were 'bad role models'. They felt just as judged in their bodies as I did in mine. In a culture obsessed with how women look after giving birth, there are no winners. It's a time we should be focusing on healing, surviving on little sleep, and getting to grips with being someone's whole entire world twenty-four hours a day, seven days a week. We shouldn't have to worry about how our bodies look to others.

With all of this going on in the background, it's no wonder so many women feel a deep sense of dissatisfaction after birth when they look in the mirror. It's yet another confidence kicker. If you're reading this while you're in recovery, I promise you – it just takes time. You *will* feel like yourself again. In the meantime, buy yourself a couple of comfortable but cute outfits that fit the body you have right now.

Because the truth is, how our bodies look after birth is just the tip of the iceberg when it comes to recovery. Don't get me wrong – getting dressed and finding clothes to wear was a nightmare, and I did want to recognise myself in the mirror. But more than anything, I just wanted my body to *work* again.

And that's where the real postnatal recovery conversation needs to happen.

After giving birth, we can expect to be discharged within twenty-four hours if things go as expected. I was sent home five hours after having Alfie, which still blows my mind.

We are then assigned appointments with a midwife or health visitor over the next two weeks. With Alfie, I had two home visits, but, with my daughter, there was one visit in clinic three days after my C-section – they were too short-staffed to provide any further care. Job done! Or not. At the magical six-week mark, we're supposed to be signed off by a doctor as suitably healed and ready to return to normal life, more or less. With both of my children, that appointment actually came at eight weeks, and the focus was far more on checking the baby than me. I was asked if I'd considered contraception ('Sex hasn't exactly been a focus, if I'm honest – BECAUSE I'M SCARED OF THE STITCHES IN MY VAGINA'). When I asked someone to check said stitches, I was told it wouldn't be necessary. No need to go anywhere near the disaster site. We're always asked if we're okay mentally, but only in a very, let's get a move on, tick-list kind of way. After that, health visitors step in, but their role is primarily focused on the baby's development, not on the mother's recovery. When I had Alfie, I never even saw a health visitor; we were one of the many families who fell through the cracks of a creaking system that is failing mums and babies.

I once text the care number about a horribly itchy rash that had spread across my breastfeeding boobs. I received a reply back a whole week later, by which point I'd already tried (and failed) to get a GP appointment. When I called the surgery, I got a phone call back from a doctor – a far quicker, but obviously deeply impersonal, way to communicate with the healthcare service. He asked me if I could send him a photo of my boobs, adding, 'although you probably don't want to do that, do you?' and then suggested I try a topical cream. When I asked if the cream was breastfeeding-friendly, he replied nonchalantly, 'Oh, good point, I don't think so actually!' Right.

In desperation, I paid for a consultation with a private dermatologist and, £300 later, I was finally prescribed a treatment that worked. I couldn't stop thinking about the millions of mothers who wouldn't be able to afford that. How can we be okay with letting women down like this? What about the women who don't have the language to advocate for themselves, or who are vulnerable for other reasons after giving birth? Where is their safety net?

In the UK it's not just that we're not supported, we can actively be harmed by the lack of care. Take the appointment (my six-week-which-was-actually-eight-week check) when my doctor told me that I could return to exercise – without a physical examination, of course. I couldn't wait to run again, so Alf and I set off into our local park. I even filmed a clip and posted it on Instagram, proudly declaring that I'd just been given the sign-off! My private pelvic health physio Marta saw and rang me. 'Ashley, please don't run until you've come to see me!'

During her physical check, she discovered I had a rectocele.

'A what? Sorry?' I had never heard this word before. Not in my birth classes, or from my midwife, or at the six-week-which-was-actually-eight-week check. If I hadn't had a social media following or the ability to afford private healthcare, I might never have known I'd sustained a birth injury. And more to the point, what damage might I have done to myself by continuing to run?

For those of you who don't know, a rectocele is a type of pelvic prolapse where your rectum pushes into the vaginal wall. It happens when the connective tissue between the rectum and vagina (the rectovaginal septum) becomes weakened or stretched. There's a lot of misinformation out there, and I've even heard from women that doctors have told them it's impossible to prolapse after birth because they're too young, that it only happens to elderly women, but this is just not true. Birth is one of the main causes of pelvic organ prolapse. Approximately half of all women experience some form of pelvic organ prolapse, and yet so many of us don't even know what it is. It's treated like a dirty secret, so many of us carry that shame alone. We deserve so much better. We should be empowered with knowledge about our bodies and supported so we can make a full recovery. I don't want to talk about any other form of 'bouncing back' if the system is ignoring our basic health and dignity. Sometimes these prolapses will improve as the body heals, especially in the early postpartum months. But often they don't just 'go away' and this is where the silence becomes harmful. Women are rarely told what to look out for, and many doctors don't screen for prolapse at the six-week check. Shockingly, lots of doctors don't even recognise the signs when women *do* come in for help.

The reason that it's important to know what's actually going on 'down there' before going back to exercise is that the repeated downward force of running can drastically cause a prolapse to worsen over time. MY VAGINA OR RECTUM COULD LITERALLY HAVE DROPPED BETWEEN MY LEGS because I went back to exercise without a physical check . . .

Here's a thought: why don't we talk about how we can get my internal body parts to bounce back in?

I know this stuff is scary. The idea that our genitals could be damaged or deformed is terrifying, especially because the world has made us believe that our value lies in having a tight and 'functioning' vagina. We may fear we'll lose our partners or never find love again. What man would want a woman with a broken vagina? We might worry we won't be able to have more children, that we'll never be desirable again. You can go overnight from feeling like an attractive woman (*GQ* Woman of the Week, no less!) to feeling broken and revolting. Imagine the impact that can have on your confidence.

The lack of education doesn't just leave us (and our partners) unprepared, it feeds a culture that expects women to disappear into motherhood with a smile and a flat stomach.

Despite the societal narrative that women are weak, and calling someone a 'pussy' insinuates a lack of strength, giving birth, whether vaginally or via C-section, is one of the most physically intense experiences any human body can go through. So why is 'grow a pair' still considered the ultimate sign of might? I've yet to see a man give birth out of his balls. Postpartum recovery is not just about pushing a baby out and losing weight (it's really, really not), and society does an injustice to us all by shifting the focus onto how we look while ignoring our health. Every system in the body, from our muscles, organs, bones, tissues, to our hormones, is affected by pregnancy and birth.

There needs to be more education and support for rehabilitating our diastasis recti, pelvic floors, and for the three possible different kinds of pelvic organ prolapses that many of us experience.

Probably one of the only postpartum issues that actually *is* talked about (sort of) is urinary incontinence. Even when I was younger, I remember hearing women joke about not going on trampolines after having kids because they'd probably wee themselves. It was always said with a laugh, like it was an inevitable part of becoming a mum. And, yes, it's incredibly common after childbirth. But what hardly anyone says out loud is this: it can be treatable.

For me personally, the worst postpartum symptom has been faecal incontinence. I still need surgery to fix an issue that will never heal on its own, and I'll admit that I've been putting it off. Faecal incontinence is quite simply the inability to control gas or bowel movements and, yes, it's as horrendous as it sounds. I think even worse than the actual symptoms are the fact that it remains such a *huge* taboo. No one wants to hear about this – nothing undermines the fantasy of the drug-free, natural birth than the reality that women may find themselves shitting themselves after it. The system is propped up by our vulnerability – so many women suffer in silence, so deeply, *deeply* ashamed and embarrassed. I felt like that too. But I've realised that the shame doesn't help me, or anyone else, and really the shame isn't mine. It's the system that stitched me up (incorrectly). So, I do my best to be frank, even though I know that a lot of people, both women and of course men, really don't want to hear it.

I cannot tell you how embarrassing it felt to experience this and how shocked I was when it first happened. I would be out in the park walking Alfie and I'd get into such a panic. It didn't help that I live in an area with lots of actual famous people, so you'd sometimes see paparazzi in the park – they actually took pictures of me the *day after* Alf was born and an online newspaper published them. I hadn't even told many people I'd had him at that point, and I suddenly started getting lots of congratulatory messages. That aside, just imagine how terrifying it is to shit yourself and then have to try and make your way home without being photographed. How humiliating it is to tell your partner to walk behind you because you'd had an accident. Understandably, it can affect a woman's willingness to go out, exercise, or be intimate. It can undermine your confidence on so many levels and the emotional toll can be huge. Had I known this wasn't normal, I might have realised something was wrong sooner instead of thinking that this was just part of it, one of those unspoken things that women just accept.

I know there are many more postpartum realities that women face, but what I want to underline yet again is that there are far more important things happening in our bodies than whether or not we can 'bounce back' in six weeks.

I think I can say with total objectivity that postnatal care in the UK is absolutely horrific. Pelvic health support is not automatically provided here unless a woman has had severe tearing or ongoing complications and, even then, access to pelvic floor physiotherapy is patchy at best with long waiting times. It's basic, overstretched and underfunded, especially when we compare it to the care received in so many other neighbouring countries, such as Holland or France. In France, all women are offered free pelvic floor physiotherapy (*rééducation périnéale*) after birth, regardless of how they delivered. They also provide postnatal home visits by midwives (called *sages-femmes*) and place a much stronger emphasis on maternal recovery as a public health priority.

My sister lived in Holland when she gave birth to her second baby, and a *kraamzorg* came to live in her home for two weeks after the birth. 'What does she do?' I asked, dumbfounded. 'Anything we need,' my sister explained. She helped with housework, looking after the toddler, and even reminding her what day her milk would come in. Needless to say, my sister didn't need to torment herself over breastfeeding this time around as she was given support and guidance. She also found it easier to care for both her newborn and toddler because she wasn't under the insane pressure to do it all herself. The *kraamzorg* is covered by basic health insurance – for women rich and poor – and is there to take pressure *off* new mothers, not pile it on.

I'll be honest, my feminine rage began to reignite during this time – like embers catching the wind. Why are we still dicking around with talk of belly fat when the real symptoms – the leaking, the tearing, the prolapse, the fear of going to the toilet – are still considered TMI? When women feel like they have to hide the truth, it doesn't lead to better care. It doesn't allow society to show us empathy. It doesn't make women less scared or less likely to experience postpartum depression. In fact, it leaves women isolated, ashamed and convinced they're the only ones who've been broken.

I honestly didn't care if I ever lost the 'baby weight', I just wanted to be able to live my life without shitting myself. But no one talks about that. Instead, we keep judging postpartum women by how they look, and not how they function or feel. And unless mothers say how wonderful it all is, we expect them to be quiet. *'Don't scare pregnant women!'*, *'Mums are so negative!'*, *'Positive birth stories don't make as good stories . . .'*

So, what do I think we should be pushing for? What are the solutions?

Well, first of all, antenatal classes — especially the ones provided by the NHS — should be straightforward and frank with us. We wouldn't be given medication without being informed of the side effects; we wouldn't be wheeled into theatre for even a minor operation without being talked through potential complications. We are not children. As long as you tell us how you'll help mend us afterwards, we can cope with it.

Post-birth, every mother deserves routine pelvic physiotherapy as standard care, and reassurance that things like incontinence and prolapse are common, usually treatable, and nothing to be ashamed of. We already know it makes financial sense in the long term, as so many health conditions later in life are linked to pelvic dysfunction. It's a no-brainer.

Postpartum bodies deserve time, rest and proper support — not pressure to squeeze back into tight jeans or conform to unrealistic ideals. And everyone in society needs to understand the scale of what a postpartum body has been through. The shame and secrecy need to go, because this culture of silence helps no one, and it certainly doesn't help improve the system for future mothers.

MILF
mɪlf

noun

Acronym for 'Mother I'd Like to Fuck', a term used to describe a sexually attractive older woman, typically one with children. While some women have reclaimed it playfully, it originated in male-dominated spaces like porn and teen movies (see: *American Pie*) as a way to objectify mothers who are seen as 'off-limits'. The MILF is fetishised precisely because she is a mother – viewed as experienced, mature and sexually transgressive. It plays into the idea that a mother would usually no longer be considered sexually desirable to men.

Male equivalent: DILF ('Dad I'd Like to Fuck') is sometimes used, but lacks the same cultural weight, aggression or objectifying tone. MILF has been mainstreamed through porn, while DILF remains niche and often affectionate.

The MILF label both hypersexualises and erases women, reducing them to a punchline, porn category or conquest. It reinforces the idea that a woman's body is only valuable through the lens of male desire – even after motherhood.

47.
Lie Back and Think of England

Before I had children, I would confidently declare that my relationship would never suffer. My worst nightmare was ending up in one of *those* relationships where you're together but not madly in love – a partnership of companionable convenience but zero passion. I swore I'd always keep the romance alive, no matter what. If my time being single taught me anything, it's that life is far too short to spend it with someone who doesn't make you happy or set your soul on fire.

I'd always been incredibly affectionate with Tommy. One of his love languages is physical touch, and he often told me that one of his favourite things about our relationship was how affectionate I was with him. It's probably worth reminding you here that we didn't live together until lockdown. It's obviously *much* easier to be romantic and touchy-feely with someone when you only see them a few times a week, on your own terms. Still, I was determined not to let the passion fade after having a baby.

What I hadn't accounted for was how scared I would feel in my own body and how utterly 'touched out' I would be. When I was asked about contraception at my six-week check, it made me feel like sex should already be back on the table. Of course, I understand the need to communicate that postpartum women can be extremely fertile, even when breastfeeding, but for the vast majority of us, contraception won't be front of mind. It's hard to feel sexy when you're genuinely scared your vagina might rip open again – especially when no one's even checked if your stitches have healed. It's hard to feel confident in your body when you're worried you might pee yourself (or worse). The question carried this invisible pressure, like I *should* be thinking about sex again. But I wasn't. I didn't feel ready. Not even close.

My nipples were still leaking, I was still sprinting home from the park to avoid shitting myself, the inside of my bum felt like it was on the outside, and I could barely stay awake, let alone muster the energy to feel horny. Postpartum hormonal changes affect libido and sexual comfort, which some believe is nature's way of helping us space out pregnancies to give mothers' bodies a chance to recover.

It's recommended that mothers leave an eighteen-month gap before getting pregnant again regardless of whether they've had a C-section or a vaginal birth. Eighteen months, not six weeks. Yet I worried a lot about what that meant. Would Tommy leave me in a fit of masculine rage? Would people whisper that I'd let myself go? That I hadn't given my partner the attention he deserved, so he had every right to look elsewhere? Would I ever feel sexy again?

Weeks turned into months, and I still didn't feel ready. Not even at three months. I think we tried once around the seven-month mark, although not because I suddenly felt ready, but because I felt so much pressure (not from him, I should add). It was uncomfortable. Painful, even. I tried to hide it, but then Tommy heard me sobbing.

The truth was, I felt like I should do it. Like it was part of being a good partner. And then he said something I'll never forget: 'You know I was there when you gave birth, right? I *saw* what happened. Do you not think I'm scared of hurting you too?' It was the first time I truly considered things from his perspective – the very human fear he might be carrying. The patriarchy teaches us that the most important thing in a relationship is to keep our man satisfied, and that if we don't, he'll discard us. But not all men are arseholes and my conversation with Tommy lifted a lot of the pressure.

Still, more time passed. And I couldn't help but notice that celebrities and influencers who'd had babies around the same time as me were already announcing second pregnancies. Was there something wrong with me?

And, honestly, there was, I just didn't know what. I couldn't even insert a tampon without pain. Every time we tried to have sex, I'd end up in tears. It was unbearable, and it took me straight back to that forced internal check just before Alfie was born.

I needed the pain to stop. I couldn't imagine feeling this way for the rest of my life. I felt damaged and like my body had betrayed me. I wanted to book a doctor's appointment, but I couldn't face stepping back into that hospital. I was also overdue for my cervical screening; I kept getting the reminder letters, which only added to the pressure. 'Ashley, if you don't go in, you might die of cancer. And you'll definitely keep living with this pain,' I'd think to myself. Eventually, I booked an appointment with one of the top gynaecologists in the country; a doctor recommended by a famous friend. If anyone could give me answers, it was him. Or so I thought.

I was nervous, but because it wasn't a hospital setting it made it feel more manageable. I told myself to put on my big girl pants – or rather, take them off.

I lay on the bed, legs apart, trying not to think about my birth. The good news? The stitches had healed well. There was nothing visibly wrong. But that was also the bad news. There was nothing visibly wrong. 'It's all in your head,' he told me. 'Okay,' I said, pulling my clothes back on. 'But how do I get it *out* of my head?' He had no answers. All that money, and I was still none the wiser. At least I could rule out cervical cancer.

Once again, my pelvic-health physio Marta came to my rescue. I told her about the pain, and within two minutes she'd figured out what was wrong. In another five, she'd already treated it. I had vaginismus, yet another condition I'd never heard of. Vaginismus is when the muscles around the vagina involuntarily tighten or spasm, making any kind of penetration, like sex, tampons, or even a cervical exam, painful or even impossible. It's the body's way of protecting itself, often in response to trauma or fear. While it's a physical condition, it's also deeply connected to emotional memory, usually your body remembering something your mind might be trying to move on from.

Marta did an internal massage, a form of manual release that gently relaxes and re-trains the muscles. The moment she said the word 'vaginismus', everything clicked into place. I wasn't crazy. And, most importantly, it wasn't in my head. What upset me the most wasn't just that I'd lived with this pain for nearly two years, it was that one of the country's leading gynaecologists couldn't recognise what was wrong. Instead of saying, 'I'm not sure, but let's explore it,' he'd told me it was all in my head. Yet another reminder of that Gender Pain Gap.

Painful sex aside, there's another unexpected part of postpartum intimacy that no one really prepares you for: the feeling of being totally and utterly 'touched out'. I've felt it since I became a mum, and I honestly don't know when that feeling will subside. Feeling 'touched out' is when you've been physically needed by small humans all day, and you feel physically overstimulated. Your body stops feeling like yours as it becomes a snack bar, a mattress, a safe place, an emotional anchor. By the end of the day, the thought of someone else touching you – even someone you love – can feel suffocating. It's not about love or attraction, but there's just nothing left to physically give.

That first year of motherhood, I was juggling everything: brutal sleep deprivation, breastfeeding on demand, working through it all because I didn't take maternity leave (if I had, I probably wouldn't have had a career to return to). I was trying to keep my head above water while keeping a tiny human alive. Then, before I knew it, there was another baby. More sleepless nights, more joy, more love. But also . . . even more people needing 110 per cent of my attention, my affection, my body.

When people talk about mums 'choosing' their kids over their partner, I get it now. It's not rejection, it's survival. We can't be everything to everyone. We're trying to do our jobs, be present with our children, stay connected to our friends, stay on top of the relentless cooking, cleaning and laundry, and somehow still feel sexy at the end of it all. It's not just exhausting, it's impossible.

I can't start my day at 5:30 a.m., get both children up and out the door, work all day, pick them up, read *The Gruffalo* for the hundredth time, cook dinner, clean up and then, in the one quiet moment I have to myself, somehow summon up the energy for sex. Most nights, if I'm not working late, I pick pyjamas and a beige snack on the sofa over anything else. Since becoming a mum, intimacy has dropped so far down my list of priorities it's basically in the basement. Not because I don't love Tommy, but because I'm burned out. Intimacy takes energy, and energy is a currency I haven't had in abundance for a long time. It's not just about sex. I don't even really want to be hugged or even touched. My kids lie with me every night, running their hands over my face and twiddling my fingers, so the moment they're finally asleep, I feel like I've hit capacity. I need my body back. My love language has gone from Physical Touch to Please Don't Touch.

That doesn't mean the spark is gone forever. It just means I've had to let go of the pressure to be everything to everyone all the time. Right now, *my children need me more*. Because I'm still navigating postpartum health issues, it feels like a mountain to climb. Perhaps if the care were better, we *would* feel better in our bodies. If we had more support so that every day didn't feel an impossible juggle of keeping up with everything, we might actually have space to feel like ourselves again.

Despite how I feel, I do feel overwhelmingly guilty and that I'm failing at being a good partner. What I've learned through this whole experience is how important it is to communicate how you feel. Even when it's awkward. Even when staying quiet feels easier. Because if you keep saying 'I'm fine' when you're actually one nudge away from tears, it builds resentment – on both sides. I understand now why so many relationships struggle in these early years of parenting. So much is changing: your identity, your time, your energy, your physical self. And there's barely any room to process it, let alone prioritise your partner.

Some couples make it through that period and slowly find their way back to each other. Some don't. And I genuinely think part of the reason they lose their way is because we don't talk about this enough. We don't talk about feeling 'touched out', about the struggle to get your sexual confidence and mojo back. I often think of the women in previous generations who were expected to be everything for everyone. Who had to do all the housework, child raising, and still look immaculate every day. Did they even have a choice to say they were not in the mood, or were they just expected to 'lie back and think of England'?

It's a phrase that's often used jokingly now, but it's thought to have come from a British aristocrat, Lady Hillingdon, who wrote in her diary in 1912: *'When I hear his steps outside my door I lie down on my bed, open my legs and think of England.'*

The phrase became a symbol of how women were taught to endure sex out of duty, not desire. And even though we like to think we've moved on, the messaging still lingers. We might not be lying back for King and country anymore, but so many of us are still pushing through pain, exhaustion or emotional disconnection to be 'good partners'. Feeling guilty if we can't perform. Because somewhere, deep down, we've absorbed the belief that if we say no too often, we'll be replaced. There is still an unspoken societal pressure to keep our partners satisfied, that if we don't provide him with sex as a basic human right, he will be excused if he seeks it elsewhere. It can make you feel that if you're not prioritising intimacy, you're doing something wrong. We're not taught to expect mutual care or healing, we're taught to feel guilty for not submitting on demand. For not wanting it even if we are still in survival mode, our bodies still recovering.

It's why so many of us fake desire or go along with sex we're not ready for. Why we carry shame when we can't rebound in every area of our lives. But what if more people knew that sex often slows down for many couples after having kids? That desire can sometimes go quiet while you're deep in the trenches. Maybe we'd all have more patience? Maybe more couples would find a way through this messy, beautiful, exhausting phase without believing that something had gone permanently wrong.

48.
Daddy Day Care and the Mother of All Mental Loads

Having children didn't just change our relationship physically – it rocked the very foundations of it. Overnight, I felt we went from being equals to role-playing more traditional gender stereotypes, and this was an arrangement I couldn't have predicted, nor one I would have ever signed up for.

I'd often think back to the moment Tommy found that pregnancy test. 'We're in this together,' he promised, and I believed him. Why wouldn't we be? We both had jobs we loved, both paid our way and shared the bills. We even took turns planning dates. We were equals. So why wouldn't we be equal parents?

When the Negative Nancys told me to enjoy trips to the nail salon while I could, I'd smile and nod, but I'd be thinking, *not me*. I have an equal partner. Of course I'll be able to get my nails done! He'll look after his own baby. But I'd underestimated how much stood between us and that dream of equality, especially in a world where dads are expected back at work immediately and mums are expected to melt into domestic life. Even if your partner wants to be equal, society doesn't really allow it.

Before I go any further, I want to say that Tommy is someone I love and respect so very deeply. For the record, he is a caring and present dad to our children, and he is far more involved in managing the load of parenthood than most men (although admittedly, the bar is so low it's in hell). He's no more perfect than I am, but I want to be really clear that my frustrations are with the system and the gendered expectations placed on us all, not with Tommy. By pointing out imbalance, my aim isn't to shame any individual man, but to highlight where the shifts in power and equality take place when you have children.

Nearly everyone experiences relationship changes when they cross the bridge into parenthood, and I wish we could be more transparent about it so it wouldn't come as such a shock. Tommy is still my coelacanth, and we continue to have shared values and mutual respect. He always considers me and my happiness, and I know I can trust and rely on him. These are huge things in a relationship. When he goes away for a work trip, he makes sure I've got what I need and thinks about stocking the fridge.

But, yes, things are different now. We don't have so much to give each other at present and that's just reality. A 2019 study of 2,000 couples found a third of relationships suffer serious problems in the months following a baby's birth,[35] with a fifth breaking up for good within the first year. One of the biggest reasons behind that strain? The disproportionate split of labour.

And when things do start to unravel, the cultural narratives we're fed are wildly different depending on who's struggling. Men are told they deserve more than a partner who's 'always tired' or 'no fun anymore'. They're encouraged to seek happiness. To put their needs first. Women, on the other hand, are told to sacrifice more. To be grateful if their partner is 'a good dad', as if that cancels out the fact they feel unsupported or unseen. Our happiness is secondary – an optional extra that should come after the needs of our children, our partner, the house, the dog, and the never-ending to-do list. We must stay for the sake of the family, and if we do become single mums, the shame is on us, regardless of the reasons.

Almost as soon as Alfie arrived, I felt the shift. Tommy was amazing, he always has been, but two weeks in, he returned to work. I'd watch him lock himself in the room next door, away from the chaos. As lockdown ended, he'd squeeze in a gym session, catch up with friends, and come home to relax in our beautiful new home and enjoy time with his baby.

And I felt that stab in my chest: resentment.

I also went back to work (my first shoot was five days post-partum) out of both financial necessity and a desire to stay tethered to something that still felt like me. But I had to do it around naps, feeds, screams and exhaustion.

Meanwhile, Tommy got to sit at a desk uninterrupted, grab a nice lunch, a coffee or two, which he could consume in total silence.

When I went back to work, I was told it was too soon.

Yet when Tommy changed a nappy, he was met with gushing praise.

While the walls closed in on me, Tommy got to watch the Euros, go on stag weekends, attend weddings, and work abroad for a week. No one asked him who was looking after the baby, because everyone knew it was me. People would ask if he was 'hands on', which basically means *does he do any of the parenting?* Every time I left the house someone would ask me who was looking after the baby, or I'd get trolled online for being selfish for putting my own needs (even a need to work) above my child's.

My friends and I can all recount instances of where we have done the majority of the parenting, whether out and about or on holiday, only for people to come up and heap praise on our partners for being *such* good dads just for playing with them. It doesn't matter if we packed the cases, sorted the passports, got everything ready for the beach, and spent all day applying suncream and entertaining. Our labour is expected and invisible, but the moment dad swoops in, he's celebrated.

I often think how much more I'd enjoy being a parent if I were a dad. Instead, I felt like I'd had a baby and been transported straight back to the expectations of the 1950s. The resentment doesn't come from a lack of love – it comes from the lack of balance.

One phrase I was completely oblivious to when I became a mum was the *maternal mental load*. No one mentioned it, not even the Negative Nancys. In contrast, I think I'd probably taken on board the idea that motherhood was some kind of extended holiday, because, you know, stay-at-home mothers *don't work*. And yet every working parent I know says the same thing: *work feels like a day off compared to parenting*.

I don't think anyone can really understand the mental load until it arrives at your door, quietly, invisibly, and completely overwhelmingly. It's almost impossible to explain unless you're in it or else it sounds trivial and insignificant. Like you're being petty. The tasks sound so small when spoken aloud. Minuscule, even. Doing the food shop. Researching weaning. Looking into childcare options. Ordering summer clothes. Remembering World Book Day. Knowing their shoe size. But the cumulative weight of all of it is enormous.

And here's what they don't tell you: even when you're through the so-called 'hard' part of motherhood – the sleepless nights, the constant feeds – the mental load *never stops*. There is always something to remember, something to plan, something to solve. My brain feels like a browser with 1,000 tabs open at all times. Some are urgent, some are half-loaded, some are crashing in the background, but all of them are mine to manage. If a ball is dropped, it will be my fault.

The disproportionate burden of the maternal mental load is probably the number-one thing Tommy and I argue about. Not the big stuff, not love or parenting values or how we feel about each other. No, it's the tiny, constant, invisible checklist that *never* seems to leave *my* head. And honestly? I never signed up to be the project manager of our lives. I would never have applied for this role. I wasn't trained for it. But, somehow, here I am, carrying the weight of our household's logistics.

When I try to articulate this to Tommy, I get hit with the classic line: *'Just ask me if you need help'* or *'Write me a list'*.

WHY do I need to write the list? I am not biologically programmed to write shopping lists. I didn't go to motherhood school. I figured it out because someone had to. Why can't we just both *see* what needs doing?

This is probably where we need to talk about 'weaponised incompetence', a term that refers to someone deliberately avoiding responsibility by pretending they don't know how to do something, or by doing it badly enough that it becomes easier for someone else to take over. It's when your partner says, 'you're just better at that stuff' or 'I'll do it if you tell me exactly what to do' and, suddenly, you're managing the task *and* managing them. It may not be malicious, or even conscious, but it's effective.

Nearly every woman I know in a heterosexual relationship is wrestling with this same invisible weight. This isn't unique to parenting, and it's true that many men will step aside from household burdens with or without children. But it becomes particularly pointed the minute a baby arrives.

For me, before we had a child, our relationship felt totally equal, but then the minute we became parents I became the keeper of everything. The one in charge. The emotional centre. The CEO of logistics. The default phone-a-friend, emergency contact for every little thing.

The maternal mental load isn't just about doing all the tasks (though obviously lots of us do more than our fair share), it's about *thinking* about them, *anticipating* them, *planning* them. It's not just making dinner – it's *deciding* on the meals, *checking* what's in the fridge, remembering who's teething and who's gone off tomatoes this week. It's staying on top of the next vaccination appointment, seeing the nursery email about 'wear red day', ordering a birthday present, figuring out the school holiday camps, arranging childcare cover, replying to the nursery group chat, and making sure we don't run out of dishwasher tablets.

It's not the doing; it's the thinking that is the unravelling.

Even when the physical chores are split fairly, the *managerial role*, the tracking, the remembering, the emotional glue – tends to fall to the mother. There is often a wildly uneven split when it comes to the responsibility for keeping everything on track in many relationships: it's 0 per cent vs. 100 per cent. And that *default parent* framework is exhausting, depleting and relentless. If our nursery calls home, they call me. If there's a school form, it's assumed I'll fill it in. Doctors, teachers, babysitters, grandparents, everyone turns to the mum first. Not because fathers aren't loving or capable, but because society still positions *us* as the central hub of the household machine.

Eventually, I tried writing down all the mental load – splitting it into two columns: who *thinks* about it, and who *does* it. I went through each line with Tommy, and, to his credit, he found it eye-opening. Even the *good men* need help seeing what they've never been taught to see. Because when you write it all down, you start to see just how much is quietly sitting in your brain. And almost always, at the very bottom of the pile, is *you*.

Household tasks	Who thinks about it	Who executes it
Creating meal plans and shopping list		
Doing the weekly shop		
Cooking meals		
Coordinating family schedules and calendar		
Budgeting and managing household finances		
Organising house repairs / services		
Remembering important dates		
Ensuring sufficient supplies (cleaning/household)		
Keeping house clean and organised		
Bins and bin day		
Doing dishes/filling and emptying the dishwasher		
Managing laundry (cleaning, drying, folding, putting away)		
Scheduling appointments (doctors, dentists etc)		
Going to appointments		
Filling out forms (nursery, school, doctor)		
Remembering friends/families' milestones		

Child raising	Who thinks about it	Who executes it
Being attuned to each child's emotional wellbeing		
Mediating sibling conflict and teaching resolution		
Reading/researching relevant development books		
Encouraging/organising hobbies/interests (and ordering relevant uniform/equipment)		
Packing school/nursery bag/lunches		
RSVPing to school/nursery/parent comms (parties)		
Gift buying for kids		
Managing morning/evening routines		
Keeping track of developmental milestones		
Dressing kids		
Keeping track of seasonal clothing and ordering new clothes		
Researching/visiting schools/nurseries		
Assisting with homework/school projects		
Scheduling/attending parent/teacher meetings		
Encouraging/researching developmental skills (potty training etc)		

	Who thinks about it	Who executes it
Tracking medical appointments and health records (vaccines up to date)		
Tracking illness/administering medicine/sick days/childcare cover		
Childproofing the home and teaching safety measures		
Preparing for emergencies (having stocked first aid kit)		
Organising playdates/birthday parties/party bags		
Managing family traditions and trips/seasonal activities		

Relationship management	*Who thinks about it*	*Who executes it*
Remembering anniversary		
Organising/planning dates		

Self-care	*Who thinks about it*	*Who executes it*
Organising activities for mental and physical wellbeing		

Is it any surprise that most of us get to the end of this list (which isn't even as exhaustive as it could be) and feel like we're failing, neglecting either our relationship or ourselves? It's not that we're not coping, it's that we're carrying too much. So many women struggle to keep on top of it all as well as keeping up the same pace in the office as we did before we had children. It's almost impossible. Yet whenever you mention any of this to a partner, you'll be seen as a nag and it's all too easy to believe *you* are the problem.

Ironically, I had to pause writing this chapter to pen a letter to Aunt Lucy from *Paddington Bear,* the teddy bear that came home from nursery with Alfie over the weekend. I had to print out photos and update her on everything he'd got up to over the weekend, so the children could read it on Monday morning. It's something a lot of schools and nurseries do, and it's seen as a lovely exercise, but it's one more thing to do. Lots of men pretend all this stuff isn't happening. Tommy asked me if he could *help*, which I'm aware I'm supposed to be grateful for.

What I've realised is this isn't just about who does the laundry or cooks dinner. It's about being *seen* and acknowledged. The worst thing about the mental load isn't even the labour, it's the invisibility of it all. It's a Sisyphean struggle where no one else can even see the boulder you're pushing uphill.

Feminism has given us more choice, more opportunity and more power. But in so many homes, women are still blending the roles of primary caregiver, domestic heads of household and career woman. We've taken on more and more, but we haven't been able to step out of the old roles. Instead, we do both and berate ourselves for doing neither well. It's no wonder we're hanging on by a thread.

And we've been socially gaslit into believing that MEN are the 'heads of the house'. Yes, many men are far more involved in the labour of family life, but very few know when the nappies have run out, or which exact brand of toothpaste isn't *too spicy* for tiny fusspots.

What we need is a cultural shift. One where 'helping out' isn't framed as a favour. One where true equality doesn't just mean splitting the chores but sharing the mental load too. I had to gently train Tommy to stop saying things like: 'I did the washing for you.' No. It's *his* house. *His* mess. *His* clothes. *His* children. It's not *for me* – you're just being a functioning adult. I love to now do housework and let him know I did it to *help* him, just to highlight how ridiculous that is.

The truth is that most mothers don't choose to carry the load. We carry it because we have to. And if we talk about it, show it, share it, we can start to shift it. We don't need help. We need change.

49.
The Bake Sale with a Side of Mum Guilt

As if the mental load wasn't heavy enough, there's another invisible weight we're expected to carry without complaint: guilt.

'Do you feel guilty for leaving the kids?' is something I get asked *a lot*. It's something Tommy gets asked *never*.

One week, I was particularly busy with work, and it happened to coincide with our nursery's charity bake sale. Now, let me just say: I *love* our nursery wholeheartedly. But someone please explain to me why, the moment you become a mother, you're suddenly expected to know how to make cakes? I have never baked a day in my life. I didn't bake before kids, and I have zero intention of taking it up now that I am even more time-poor, juggling deadlines, laundry, life admin and two tiny humans. The 1950s called again and it wants its cupcakes back. No shade to the baking mums, I love that you love baking. It's just never been my jam (pun intended).

My plan was to do what I imagine many non-baking working mothers do – buy a box of cupcakes from the supermarket, slightly mash them up, throw on a few sweets, and pass them off as homemade. Except . . . I forgot to do that. I forgot the whole thing. And, to be honest, it kind of defeats the point of a charity bake sale if I spend more money on ingredients than I would just donating. Still, as I walked into the nursery and saw the lovingly decorated table of muffins and brownies, I felt that familiar stab of guilt. 'Do you take card?' I asked feebly, already cringing. I felt like I'd let the kids down. I've always been a high achiever. I hate missing the mark, even for a bake sale. So, I text Tommy: 'Do you feel guilty about missing the bake sale?' He replied: 'When is it?'

That moment, to me, sums up *mum guilt*. I was wracked with shame over not fitting a cake sale into my already overloaded brain, and he didn't even know it was happening. Of course, I'm generalising. But this is what I know: I've never once heard someone ask a dad if he feels guilty for working, or for going to the gym, or for missing nursery pick-up. But mums? We get asked *all the time*.

'Mum guilt' is a term most of us know all too well. It's that gnawing, ever-present feeling that you're not doing enough, not doing it right, or somehow falling short, whether that's in the eyes of your children, your work colleagues, or society as a whole. It creeps in over the smallest things: letting the kids watch too much TV, serving fish fingers again, missing a reading record. And then it barrels in over the big things, like choosing to go back to work, needing time for yourself, or not feeling joyful every moment of the day. But why does it cut so deeply?

I believe it's a reflection of the astronomical expectations placed on us. We are supposed to raise emotionally intelligent, healthy, independent, creative children, while also keeping the house running, excelling at our jobs (if we have one), maintaining friendships, keeping the romance alive, staying fit, cooking nutritious meals, and still having time to respond to the WhatsApp group about playdates.

Thanks to social media, we're constantly bombarded with other people's highlight reels, from homemade sensory trays, matching outfits, Bento box lunches to themed birthday parties. We're comparing ourselves not just to other mums on our street, but to curated, filtered performances of perfection from people we don't even know.

Meanwhile, dads? Dads still get standing ovations for dressing their kids in clothes that don't fit them. We applaud them for just showing up and doing their best, which is, honestly, sometimes a bit shit. That's not to say there aren't amazing, involved fathers out there. There are. And all attempts at good parenting deserve to be celebrated. But the bar has been set so differently. While mums are judged for every decision, from feeding to sleep routines to childcare, dads are still praised for *not going to the football*. The result? A double standard where mothers internalise guilt for things fathers don't even know exist. No wonder they can weather the parenthood journey so much more easily – none of this takes up real estate in their brains.

As I hope you can tell from this story, what we've learned, we can *unlearn*. Guilt thrives on perfectionism and feeds off unrealistic expectations. And the only way to shrink it is to speak about it, laugh about it, push back against it. Your children don't need a perfect mother or a Pinterest-worthy childhood. If letting them watch TV means you can catch up with the weekly shop or have a hot cuppa, then so be it. If a pouch or a ready meal saves you thirty minutes during a week you feel like you're chasing your tail, then go for it. We're not robots and we cannot do it all.

Taking time out for yourself, pursuing your passions, or forgetting a bake sale does not make you a bad mum. It makes you a whole person. Mum guilt might never go away entirely, but we can stop giving it so much power. If there's no such term as *dad guilt,* I refuse to feel guilty for not being able to split myself in two.

NAG

næg
noun

a woman who is seen as persistently complaining, criticising or asking for something, usually from a male partner. It's often used to dismiss or ridicule women's attempts to express needs, hold others accountable or manage domestic and emotional responsibilities. The term has roots in reducing women's voices to background noise, implying she is irritating, excessive and unreasonable.

Male equivalent: There's no direct male counterpart to *nag*, which is telling. When men raise concerns or give instructions, they're often seen as assertive or taking charge. But when women do the same, they risk being labelled *nags*. It reflects the imbalance in how emotional labour and communication are valued depending on gender. *Nag* trivialises the unpaid, often invisible work women do in relationships and households. It's one of many terms weaponised to silence, belittle or dismiss women, particularly in heterosexual relationships, when they dare to ask for their partner to do something in the home.

50.
Crash Landing from Cloud Nine

I'm not a religious person, but if there *is* such a thing as heaven, then, for me, it would resemble the first four months of both of my babies' lives. The moment before the birth trauma, and the tiredness and the relationship changes sink in, and it's just you and this tiny little baby with a perfect-smelling head. Your new family unit. They were truly the best months of my existence, and I know that, when I'm on my deathbed, they'll be the days I relive. I couldn't believe I had ever thought that I didn't want children! I couldn't stop staring at them! I was also in awe of my body for creating them. Watching Tommy become a dad made my love for him explode, he was just so good immediately.

I knew there was a risk of postnatal depression during the fourth trimester. My understanding was that our hormones drop after birth and that affects everyone differently. The first time around, I even ate my placenta in the hope it might keep the baby blues at bay. And whether it was placebo effect or not, it worked! I remember getting to the end of the fourth trimester and thinking: *Wow. I made it. No depression!* I know it's not like that for everyone. I saw mums around me struggling from the start: dealing with premature babies, breastfeeding challenges, reflux, or just the brutal reality of living with an infant. I felt so lucky to have escaped all that. For me, those first few months were pure magic: I was soaring. And I don't say that to romanticise motherhood, I say it to honour the joy.

Motherhood doesn't have to be negative, I'd think, *I am resilient, and I have a positive mindset.* People often talk about losing themselves in motherhood, but I felt like I found myself. For so long, I'd been chasing love – real, reciprocal love – and suddenly, here it was. My heart, outside of my body, in human form. This was everything I'd been searching for and more.

In my teens and twenties, I ignored my gut instinct constantly. But motherhood brought with it a clarity I'd never known. I know a lot of new parents doubt their abilities, but I never doubted mine. And even though, like every mother, I've felt the stab of guilt, I've always known I'm an amazing mum. And I wish all mums felt empowered to trust themselves. It might sound bonkers, but, with Alfie, I felt telepathically connected from the moment he was born. Even now, I understand his cries, his moods, his mind. And Ada? She was easy. Everything I found hard with Alf, like breastfeeding and the sleep, she just did with ease. If Alfie was my teacher, Ada was my healer.

Those first four months felt like being in a bubble – me, them, and the world on mute. Time moved differently. Days blurred into nights and nights into days as I was cocooned in love and purpose. During lockdown with Alfie, he gave my days structure and meaning. The world was scary, but he was my constant. We walked in the park, cuddled up watching movies, and just existed outside of time.

With Ada, it was the same, but different. No lockdown this time, and with a toddler in tow, it was a bit more chaotic. But I got to do all the things I missed the first time around. Lunches with friends. Binge-watching *Married at First Sight Australia* while Alf was at the childminder. (It was during those days watching fuck boy Harrison that I taught Ada all about red flags and gaslighting while she dozed on my chest.) Second time around, I knew how quickly it would pass, so I savoured every sleepy stretch, every milky sigh, every moment of her tiny body curled up against mine.

There's something sacred about those early days. It's like a portal opens, a quiet little pocket of the universe where time slows down and the only things that matter are the rhythm of your baby's breathing and the warmth of their body on your chest. I was high as a kite on love. High on oxytocin, connection and the magic of new motherhood. I was floating on cloud nine. But what goes up must come down — and when I came down, it wasn't a gentle descent.

The third UK lockdown began on 6 January 2021, three days before Alfie was born, and it wasn't until 17 May that shops reopened, and people were finally allowed to meet outside again. When that happened, I was elated. Finally, my little boy would meet our friends and family. For the first time, I could take him into shops and show him life beyond our tiny London flat. Little did I know that, as the world opened up, something inside me began to close in. It started to dawn on me how much the world as I knew it had moved on while I was sat still.

While everyone else seemed to be returning to something that resembled their old lives, I realised just how unrecognisable mine had become. The penny dropped that the pandemic had masked how totally divorced my life had become from the rhythm of the world I'd always known. I had gone into lockdown as a carefree DJ. I travelled the world, I stayed out late, I hosted dinner parties with my girlfriends, and I was incredibly independent.

I came out the other side with cracked nipples, a baby who never slept, a body I didn't recognise, and a career that felt like it had vanished without a trace. I didn't have a single DJ booking in my diary, and I felt like I'd been brushed off by every client I'd reached out to. And as I scrolled through Instagram, I saw everyone else rebuilding and flourishing. But all I had to offer were dark eye bags and mental confusion. Somewhere along the way, the old me had slipped through my fingers, and I began to feel terrified that I'd never be able to get her back. And that depression I'd thought I'd dodged started to edge its way in.

As I walked down the high street, I felt utterly alone. I had no new mum friends, and my old friends had gone back to their old lives – our old life. I had become incredibly isolated. What made that even worse was that we'd made the decision to move out of London. It made sense on a logical level: more space, better value for money. Tommy's parents lived by the seaside in Essex, and he worked in the city, so we moved somewhere in between. 'I'm self-employed,' I said. 'I can work anywhere.' Ninety minutes didn't seem that far from my friends back when I was child-free. But it turns out that ninety minutes with a baby is the equivalent of living in a different solar system. If someone invited me out at 7:30 p.m., I'd have to leave at 5:30 p.m. and wouldn't get home until midnight. I'd spend more time travelling than socialising. And Alfie couldn't be left that long anyway. If we'd still lived nearby, I could've popped out and back again if he'd needed me, but I hadn't really factored that in when we made our decision.

The weight of what I'd done started to settle on my chest. And not just the move, the whole decision to become a mother. Motherhood is one of the most irreversible decisions a person can make. You can leave a job. You can break up with a partner. You can walk away from friendships that no longer serve you. You can move house, move countries. But you can't *un*-have a baby. And as much as I loved Alfie with every fibre of my being, I felt trapped. As much as I felt ashamed for feeling that way, I did.

Was I a monster for thinking this? I'd stare at his perfect face and feel so guilty. I must be the most selfish woman on the planet. Ironically, people used to call me selfish when I said I didn't want kids. But now I felt selfish for bringing a child into my life and still yearning for the freedom of my old one. I looked around and other mums seemed to be thriving – even the ones who struggled early on. Was I the only one feeling this way? Was *this* meant to fulfil me? Why wasn't it enough?

It felt like I'd fallen for a lie that tells women that motherhood will complete us, that it's the pinnacle of female purpose. That if we struggle, we're ungrateful. I'd internalised it so deeply that even in my moments of despair, I thought *I* was the problem, not the rose-tinted story I'd been sold.

The world expects women to give everything and expect nothing. To sacrifice ourselves for our children and smile while we do it. To find joy in isolation, purpose in exhaustion, and identity in servitude. And when we can't, we're made to feel like monsters. These thoughts ate me alive. I felt trapped inside a version of life that I'd been told would make me whole.

51.
Is it Normal to Regret Motherhood?

The problem with being up *a lot* at night was that my brain was always awake. I would often scroll on my phone and look at everyone else's lives and it would compound my feelings of loneliness. My child-free friends had all moved on without me and I really missed them. I'd then watch other mums who I followed share the highlights of motherhood and I couldn't relate. I'd stare over at Tommy sleeping soundly under the duvet as I'd contort my body into increasingly uncomfortable positions with Alfie attached to my boob. Was I meant to feel so alone?

With shame, I'd search 'is it normal to regret motherhood?'. I felt like a criminal for even typing it, as if someone was going to cart me away for being so abnormal. How could I even write those words? Motherhood is like coupledom in some ways, as it's packaged as the thing that brings us total peace and contentment. I loved my baby, but I hated my life as a mum. I hated the finger puppets. I hated the lack of freedom. I hated singing 'Baby Shark'. I hated that my body didn't work. I hated that I had no DJ bookings. I hated that Tommy's life had gone back to normal. I hated that this was suddenly meant to be enough.

Regret around motherhood is probably one of the most taboo topics in society. For generations, mothers have been expected to love every moment of raising children, finding pure joy in the experience, and never questioning their decision to become parents. Happy to stay at home raising the children and fulfilling all domestic duties with a smile on their face. The work is never done and most of it is soul destroying. Mundane, repetitive, boring.

And yet we're sold it as our biological destiny. That we should be grateful. That this is what we were made for.

On top of that, a lot of the struggles we face as mums are because the system isn't made with us in mind. In fact, it's made to encourage us to stay at home for as long as possible. Whether it's the poor postnatal care, the eye-watering cost of childcare, the fact school hours don't align with work hours, the gender imbalance of domestic labour no matter what the balance of the income, the lack of paternity leave, I could go on and on. Yet if we dare mention any of these realities, admit that we're struggling to feel the *normal* feelings, we're deemed ungrateful or negative. We're told we don't love our children. This dissatisfaction is what iconic feminist author Betty Friedan labelled 'the problem that has no name' in 1963's *The Feminine Mystique*.

'What will your son think when he sees you complaining about motherhood?' people often said to me when I tried to be honest about my struggles. To this day, I always reply that hopefully he will understand what I overcame and sacrificed to raise him. Should he ever become a father, he will understand how difficult it can be. He won't be fooled by the fantasy; he won't take anything for granted and will understand that there is a multiplicity of emotion that comes when a woman has a baby. We will engage with each other in an authentic and genuine way, and I will tell him that I struggled, but my love for him got me through it.

It can be *normal* to feel regret about motherhood at times. It doesn't make you a bad mother, a bad person, or unworthy of love, it makes you human. Motherhood is an all-encompassing experience that often comes with significant sacrifices. It can feel like your identity gets erased, it totally upends your freedom, your career, your relationships, and even your mental health. It can dissolve your esteem and confidence. There would be something wrong with our sense of logic if we didn't ever think, 'Did I make the right choice?'

This feeling of regret isn't about not loving your children. Most mothers who experience regret still love their kids deeply. Instead, it's about grieving the loss of who we were or what our lives looked like before motherhood. Regret often stems from the lack of adequate support systems. Women are often left to carry the mental load of parenting alone, with little family or institutional support. This isolation can make motherhood feel not only overwhelming but deeply unbalanced. It's meant to take a village, but few of us live in one anymore. It's no wonder so many women silently question if they've made the right choice. If you've felt regret about motherhood, know this: you're not alone. At least 14 per cent of mothers will explicitly admit to having regrets at some point about having a baby,[36] and that figure is thought to represent a far higher proportion, as so many women feel unable to say it out loud even in confidential research. These feelings are far more common than society lets on, and they don't define you as a person or as a mother. What matters is the love and effort you put into your children's lives, even when it's hard.

I don't want to minimise anyone's feelings, and it is true that some women will continue to feel regret for their choice, even as they love their kids. But I can say that, for me, things got better. Today, I love my life, and I love my children, and

I don't mourn my old existence as much as I used to. There are things I still miss, of course. I miss having more disposable income, I miss lie-ins, I miss being able to do things – for work or pleasure – without having to deal with logistics. I miss doing things for myself.

When I look back, I sometimes think: would I have been happier if I'd stuck to my guns and remained child-free? I'll never know. I was happy then, and it certainly took me time to find my new happy. I cannot bear the thought that my children wouldn't exist, and they have certainly given my life a new and different sense of purpose, but I also think of it like the film *Sliding Doors*. There was joy in both versions of my life, either side of the choice. Coming to terms with that can take time and we should never be made to feel that we're abnormal or even evil if we have feelings like this.

Because we were sold a promise. A promise that motherhood would complete us. That it would give us purpose, joy, identity. And when it doesn't? We're made to feel broken. Like we failed. But maybe the problem isn't us. Maybe the problem has no name because we were never meant to speak it out loud.

52.
The Weight of it All

One Saturday when Alf was still a babe in arms, Tommy was invited to go to Twickenham with some of his family to watch the rugby. Saturday came along. 'We're meeting two hours before the game,' he told me. I did the maths. Two hours to get there + two hours pre-game drinks + two-hour game + two hours post-game drinks + two hours back = ten hours of me home alone with Alfie. After a whole week of being alone in the house with Alfie. My brain went into overdrive – I just couldn't do it.

By this point I felt so lonely I was having thoughts of suicide. I wouldn't say that I was suicidal, more that I was having suicidal ideations. My brain kept imagining me going upstairs and ending it. They weren't voluntary thoughts; they were *intrusive thoughts*. And intrusive thoughts are incredibly common after birth, especially when the lack of sleep compounds the pressure of new responsibilities. I tried to communicate how I was feeling to Tommy, and he just couldn't understand how I could be feeling the way I was. I was that self-harming teenager once again – that nuisance girl who was 'ungrateful' and 'unable to cope'.

'Please just don't go,' I said. And he didn't. Though, of course, I felt guilty about that too. As I write these words, I feel a deep sense of shame that my mental health got that low.

Especially because I'd lost my friend – the wonderful Caroline Flack – to suicide just eighteen months earlier. I mourned her loss alongside the whole nation. I watched as the world shared how important it was to be open about our mental health, and we told everyone to *be kind*. But when it was me, when *I* was the one struggling, I buried it.

That's why I feel it's so important to talk about this now. Maternal mental health is still wrapped in stigma. Too often, it's dismissed as 'hormones' or trivialised as the 'baby blues'. Yes, hormones absolutely play a part. But, in my case, it was something bigger. It was the seismic shift of suddenly being someone's entire world, twenty-four hours a day. It was the loss of my freedom, identity, career as I knew it, friendships, and even parts of my relationship.

A friend of mine spent a decade trying to conceive. She left her job before her third and final round of IVF, which was thankfully successful. She later admitted that, before becoming a mum, she would feel anger when she heard mothers speak openly about their struggles. 'How ungrateful,' she'd think. 'If I'm ever lucky enough to be a mum, I will never complain.' But after experiencing a traumatic birth (she gave birth on her own in the hospital toilet of the labour ward because medical staff told her she wasn't ready to push, then had a haemorrhage and ended up in critical care away from her baby) and the brutal reality of early motherhood, she told me she'd *never* have another child. Her story stuck with me. Because it made me realise just how many women are holding pain they feel they're not allowed to express. She was grateful AND she struggled.

Maternal mental health is *very* real. Approximately one in five women in the UK develop a mental health condition during pregnancy or within the first year postpartum.[37]

Suicide remains the leading cause of direct maternal deaths between six weeks and one year after childbirth. But even with all this, only about 10 per cent of new mothers receive any kind of support. And many don't seek help at all, silenced by a fear of being judged.

We have to change this.

Women shouldn't have to break in silence. They shouldn't have to feel *grateful* instead of *struggling*. They shouldn't have to whisper about the weight they're carrying.

Because this isn't just about individual women.

It's about how society treats mothers.

And it's time we did better.

53.
Finding Your Pink

I am so happy to say that I made it through that horrific period of my life. And truthfully? I'm *glad* I went through it. As painful as it was, it reshaped me. Like all struggles, it stretched my heart and my capacity for empathy. It made me softer in the ways that matter, and fiercer in the ways that count. I care deeply about new mums now, *even* (and maybe especially) the ones who, like I once was, are still floating in that blissful newborn bubble. I never try to pop their joy. I marvel at it. I smile with them. And, quietly, I make sure they know I'm here. That if their bubble ever bursts, even if it's months down the line, I'll be waiting on the other side, no judgement, just open arms.

There wasn't one big, dramatic moment that turned everything around for me. No magical fix or perfect formula. But there were glimmers. Kindnesses. Acts of love that helped me rise slowly from the ashes.

One big shift that turned the dial was admitting that we'd made a miscalculation. The move out of London had been sensible on so many levels, but it turned out to be the totally wrong choice for our family. So, in the opposite direction to most thirty-something parents, we made the decision to move *back* into London. That changed everything. Re-finding myself in the city brought something back to life inside me. I got to be spontaneous again. I could put the kids to bed, pop round to a friend's house at 7:30 p.m., laugh over a glass of wine, and still be home and in my PJs by 10. That kind of freedom felt radical. I was surrounded by girlfriends once more, by energy, by life.

I've never really felt like I fit in anywhere – but maybe that's why London suits me. Most people here are from somewhere else. It's the only place that has ever truly felt like home. That might change one day. But, for now, moving back gave me something precious: a tribe. Before long, I found the kind of mum friends you'd be friends with even if you weren't a mum. Women who get what you're going through but don't just talk about their kids. Women who reminded me who I was. Living closer to work meant less time commuting and more time living, and life got less lonely.

But if I had to pinpoint the biggest factor, I would say it was mainly time passing. Healing came gradually. Slowly, I started to feel like myself again – maybe not the *same* self, but an evolved version of who I once had been. Someone more layered.

Eventually, we decided to invest in childcare for Alfie, which came with its own logistical circus. But it also meant I could focus on my work again. I still remember the moment of *elation* I felt as the door to the childminders closed, Alf safely inside. I went home, opened my laptop, hot coffee in hand. Just getting to work in silence without distraction felt magical. *Just me.* I almost couldn't believe it.

I know lots of mums hate going back to work and feel guilty about their child being in childcare, but it wasn't like that for me. Having time to focus on work allowed me to stop feeling like a failure in both parts of my life – when I was juggling both I couldn't be a good mum, nor could I do my work well. Now when I saw Alfie I could be fully present with him. Truthfully, you have to find what works best for you and there isn't a template for that. Through the positive experience I had with Alfie, I stopped holding myself to unrealistic standards and didn't hesitate to carve out space for myself to work the second time around. Ada started in childcare at six months. I know that saved my sanity and probably months of drowning, and I had seen what that looked like. I was never going back there again.

Another huge helping hand in my journey was discovering the term that changed everything for me: matrescence. I quite literally cried when I first read about it. Finally, *language* for what I was feeling. It was like someone had handed me a map through the wilderness I'd been wandering through. *This* was what I'd been experiencing. Not failure. Not weakness. Not madness.

First coined by anthropologist Dana Raphael in the 1970s, 'matrescence' describes the physical, emotional, hormonal, psychological and social transformation a woman undergoes as she becomes a mother. Just like adolescence, it marks a subtle space, a *becoming*, a reshaping of identity. While adolescence is widely recognised, supported, and even expected, matrescence is mostly invisible. Undiscussed. Dismissed. Sound familiar?

Matrescence isn't something you 'bounce back' from. It doesn't follow a neat timeline. It can take months or even years. I'd say my own path there took about two years, but, by that point, I'd had another baby. So, it's taken a long time to find my confidence in myself again and feel like ME. I suppose we can describe it as the reconciliation between the 'old' you and the 'new' you. It's about grieving who you were, while learning to love who you're becoming. About squaring the tenderness you feel for your baby with the ache of everything you've let go of.

Matrescence can bring joy and clarity and beauty in the moment. It can also bring an overwhelming sense of purpose. But it can also come with confusion, rage, sadness and loss. And until I found a name for it, I was left believing only I had these thoughts, when in fact, they're signs we're *changing*. To varying degrees, lots of these emotions are universal.

When I learned about matrescence, I realised I wasn't broken. Instead, I was in transition, like a butterfly. Transitions are hard, exhausting and physically and emotionally depleting. They require compassion, patience and community. Just knowing the word 'matrescence' allowed me to name what had once felt invisible.

It was also around this time that I learned that flamingos lose their pink colour when they become parents. The demands of raising their young are so intense that their vibrant, signature colour fades. Over time, as their babies grow, they slowly get their colour back. That hit me so hard. Because that's exactly how it felt: like the colour had drained from my world, from *me*. But slowly, gently, I began to find it again. Through getting to focus on my work. Through getting a good night's sleep. Through getting to spend time with my friends. Through getting to be Ashley James and not 'just a mum'. It was having conversations with people again that didn't centre around babies or sleep schedules. I had lost my pink, but slowly it came back to me and now I would say that it is brighter than ever because it carries both the joy and pain of everything I battled through. It's a confidence that has steel at its core. My new pink is far kinder and more understanding, both of children and mothers. It no longer upholds misogynistic views about any women – whether they are a mum or child-free.

I now know that motherhood doesn't erase us, we're still in there. We just need time and support to get our colour back and find our pink again. And that will happen, even if it takes some of us a bit longer to get there.

Let me say this clearly: for as long as we tell mothers to be grateful while failing to understand matrescence, we risk failing them completely. We need to stop shrinking mothers into labels and instead expand our compassion. Support is not just a nicety, it's a necessity. Through every identity shift, every bodily change and every relationship test, we need to offer more than judgement and unsolicited advice. We need to stop brushing off the systemic lack of support as a negative mindset and instead offer solidarity.

54.
The Power of Mum

For all the difficulties, challenges and expenses that come with motherhood, it's also blasted my heart wide open. If my single chapter made me realise that life is short and for living, motherhood has taught me that I want to live a long life and savour every moment with my children. In so many ways, my purpose and drive are now for them. I look forward to waking up and seeing their faces (although I wish it wasn't quite so early), and I run home from work hoping I get to pick them up or see them before they fall asleep.

I still lie in bed with both of my children every night. I read stories to them both from Alfie's big bed and I lie beside them until they are safely dreaming. What a privilege to be someone's whole entire world. To be their favourite person, their safety net and their home. One day they will look at me with all my imperfections. They will recognise my flaws and talk about all the things I didn't do right. But, today, I am their everything.

If motherhood has taught me anything, it's that no one else has the answers. There is no single right way to do this. There is only *your* way. And the sooner we stop searching for flawlessness and start trusting our own instincts, the freer we become. We don't need permission to do things differently. We don't need to apologise for protecting our peace or choosing what works best for *our* family. We are allowed to find it hard. We are allowed to love it. We are allowed to feel both of those things in the same breath. That is what confidence as a mother looks like.

The myth of the perfect mum was never built *for* us, it was built to keep us too busy, too tired, too self-critical to ask for more. It thrives on guilt and comparison and serves only to rob us of the self-belief that is so often in short supply in our brand-new job role. But when we stop judging each other and start really supporting one another, something powerful happens. We reclaim the option of doing things our own way.

If the last few years have schooled me on anything, it's just how incredible mums are. Not just the ones who do it like me, but *all* of them. We truly are the backbone of society and always have been. I am in awe of the single mums. Truly. How society ever let us shame you is beyond me. You stayed. You showed up. You kept going when there was no one to tag in, when the night was long, and the energy was gone. You deserve all the praise and support the world has to give. I'm constantly inspired by stay-at-home mums too. You do the unpaid, unseen work of raising tiny humans and I never want to hear you tell anyone that you 'do not work'. It's round-the-clock caregiving, emotional labour and relentless routines with little rest. You ARE working, and that work is important. And to the working mums – I see you too. I *feel* you. Balancing deadlines and dinner time, meetings and medicine doses. Trying to be present in two places at once and constantly feeling like you're falling short in both. You're not. You're holding so much in your heart and head and you're doing it with grit, grace and, often, not enough credit.

To the married mums who feel like single mums because your partner sleeps through the night feeds or heads off to golf while you're scraping together the energy to survive the day, you're not imagining it. That mental load you're carrying? It's real. And it's heavy, and unless you have explicitly chosen to shoulder it alone, it shouldn't be your exclusive burden. To every mum who is grieving, recovering, rebuilding, or just getting through the day, you're not failing. Motherhood isn't one path. It's a thousand different ones, all of them messy and meaningful and worthy of respect. So, whatever yours looks like, I hope you know this: you're more than enough.

As I reflect on all of this, what I've learned, what I've let go of, what I've reclaimed, there's something else I want to say. Parenthood didn't just change me as a woman. It changed my relationship too. In many ways, it ripped it apart and remade it as something new. We're still navigating the waves of those changes, still trying to find our way to this fresh partnership. And yet what remains, what's always been there, is love, respect and the shared knowledge that we are both *brilliant* parents.

The truth is, the only reason I am able to thrive in my career, able to have a social life, able to write the words in this book, is because I have a partner who fully shows up as a father. Who doesn't just 'help', but also *parents*. Who doesn't see my success as a threat to his own, but as something we are building together. Who does the dishwasher every day, and who takes the washing out so that I don't forget about it. I may have had to teach him that he is not 'helping', but he is right at the coal face with me.

That should be the expectation, not the exception. Because when fathers show up fully, it doesn't just lighten the load, it changes the narrative. It models a new kind of equality, one that doesn't live in theory, but in the everyday.

So, as this chapter closes, I hope you walk away with one message above all: *trust your gut*. Your instincts are wise, so have confidence in them. You know what's best for you and your children, even when the world tries to convince you otherwise. I would love for you to walk away with more compassion too. For yourself, but also for other mums doing it differently.

That's why the next bit matters. Because while motherhood lives in our homes and hearts, the conditions that shape it – childcare, healthcare, housing, work, safety – are political. In fact, the personal has always been political. So, let's keep going. Use your votes wisely! Let's take this fire and turn it outward. Because if we want to change the world our children grow up in, we have to change the systems we're raising them within.

55.
Being a Boy Mum

This book is about womanhood, but I can't talk about women without also talking about boys. Arguably, one of the most important roles in my life now is being a boy mum. I'm raising my son, Alfie, in a world that is trying to teach him a very narrow definition of manhood. It's a world where toxic masculinity is normalised, where violence is rewarded, and where sensitivity is mistaken for weakness. It's a world where the internet is flooded with male influencers who preach hate, dominance and misogyny, with their messages designed to turn back the clock and undo feminism reaching millions of boys just like mine.

While I worry for my daughter, I worry just as much for my son. Alfie is a sweet, kind, sensitive little boy. He loves cuddles. He enjoys dressing up as Elsa from *Frozen*. He plays with dolls and notices when someone is sad. He embraces his friends and says 'I love you' without hesitation or shame. I look at him and feel so proud of who he is, but I also wonder how I can protect that softness in a world that will doubtless try to harden it.

And that's what this book is about: the labels, expectations and boxes. And the damage they do to our sense of self. We talk a lot about how women are boxed through labels such as 'slut', 'prude', 'bossy', 'frumpy'; but the undeniable truth is that boys and men are boxed in too. Any boy who doesn't fit the rigid, narrow mould of what a man is 'meant' to be: stoic, straight, strong, dominant, is labelled and 'othered'. Especially if they're soft. Or sensitive. Or queer. These aren't just words. They're warnings. Be less like that. Be more like this. Or else.

This narrow, rigid and often violent version of masculinity we see glorified in our culture is harmful and is often referred to as toxic masculinity. This term has been twisted by some to suggest that men aren't allowed to be men anymore, but that's not what it means at all. Toxic masculinity doesn't mean that masculinity is inherently bad, but rather that these rigid, performative rules around it harm not just women and girls but also men and boys. It teaches them that they shouldn't cry, that they shouldn't show emotion, that asking for help is a weakness. It suggests that real power lies in dominance, not empathy, and that to be respected, they must be feared. It encourages men to disconnect from their feelings, which in turn disconnects them from themselves and from others. It also frames femininity as feeble, which not only devalues women but teaches boys that any traits associated with girls, such as sensitivity, kindness and cooperation need to be suppressed. These emotions aren't gendered, they make us human, and we are setting boys up to unlearn their humanity.

And it's dangerous. The consequences of these messages are not abstract; they are devastatingly real. In the UK, a woman is killed by a man every three days.[38] Gender-based violence has been declared a national emergency, and yet we continue to treat it as an unfortunate series of unrelated incidents, rather than as the cultural epidemic it really is. If violence on this scale were committed systematically based on race or religion, we would not hesitate to call it extremism or terrorism. But when it's committed by men against women, we're still met with defensiveness and dismissal. We hear 'not all men' more often than we hear 'what can we do to change this?'

Meanwhile, a dark online culture continues to grow, often referred to as the 'manosphere'. This includes a network of forums, influencers and social media platforms where misogyny is dressed up as self-improvement. Male figures offer boys a version of masculinity that is built on control, entitlement and dominance. They frame women as property and emotions as weakness, and they do so with charisma, confidence and reach. These men are not on the fringes. They're viral. They're mainstream. They're being welcomed onto global platforms and into conversations with world leaders.

One of the most dangerous aspects of this online world is the rise of 'incel' culture, short for 'involuntary celibate'. What began decades ago as a term to describe male loneliness has evolved into an ideology rooted in entitlement and rage. Many of these men believe that women owe them attention, sex and love and, when they don't receive it, they blame women, feminism and an imagined loss of male power. These communities don't just share frustration; they breed hate. They have been directly linked to acts of real-world violence, including mass shootings. Security experts now recognise incel ideology as a terrorism threat. The UK government acknowledged in a 2023 study that incel forums are influencing boys and men here in Britain and yet they continue to grow. And, still, we're not talking about them enough, certainly not with our children.

What's particularly frightening is that these spaces don't start out with blatant hate. They start with isolation. They appeal to insecurity and a lack of confidence. They draw boys in with promises of self-esteem and belonging. They sell misogyny as masculinity. They offer boys an identity, and, for too many, it works. Because in a world that mocks male vulnerability and sees female confidence as a threat, what else are we offering them?

That's where we come in. As parents, carers, educators and adults who shape the world our children grow up in, we have a responsibility to show our boys that there is another way to be. A better way. We need to provide them with real-life role models who demonstrate that kindness, vulnerability and emotional intelligence are not only acceptable but are essential. We need men who show up. Who listen. Who admit when they're wrong. Who share the load at home without needing to be asked or applauded. Men who raise their sons with care and awareness. Men who understand that masculinity can – and should – include gentleness, empathy and softness. We cannot leave this work to mothers alone.

Boys are watching all of us and they are learning not just from what we say but from what we do. They notice what we tolerate in relationships. They notice who does the school run. Who apologises. Who cooks dinner. Who gets interrupted. Who is listened to. They absorb how we treat each other and how we allow ourselves to be treated. If we want to raise better men, we must model better ways of being. We must show them that love is not weakness and that crying is not shameful. That leadership doesn't require cruelty. That equality is not a threat. That female confidence is the goal. We must raise them with boundaries and freedom, with love and accountability. We must talk to them early on about consent, respect, emotions and power. We must teach them that jokes that punch down aren't funny, and that no always means no. We must remind them that feminism isn't about undermining men, it's about lifting *everyone* up.

This isn't just about keeping girls safe. It's about giving boys the freedom to be their full authentic selves. It's about dismantling a culture that robs them of their empathy. So, I will continue to raise Alfie with love, with care. I will follow his curiosity about things without shaming him. I will let him be gentle and allow him to cry. I will teach him to apologise and to listen and to take responsibility for his actions. I will show him that strength and tenderness can coexist – that doing something 'like a girl' carries just as much worth as doing it 'like a boy'. And I will do everything in my power to protect that softness for as long as I can, while preparing him to be the kind of man who protects it for himself, and for others. Because the next generation depends on boys who grow into good men. And they deserve the chance to live beyond the labels too.

ELDERHOOD

HAG

hæg

noun, offensive

a derogatory term used to describe an old woman, typically one who is perceived as unattractive, unpleasant or witch-like. The word is rooted in misogyny and ageism, often used to dehumanise, mock or diminish women as they age and lose perceived sexual or social value.

Male equivalent: There is no direct male equivalent with the same level of vitriol or social consequence. The closest equivalent might be *codger*, which while derogatory is far more a term of affection or mild derision. It could also be compared with *silver fox*, which has connotations of power, attractiveness and shows how age can elevate a man's perceived social worth.

As we reach the present day, and as the words of this book come to a close, it's worth noting that, of course, my story isn't finished. I'm thirty-eight years old, and even though I feel like I've lived multiple lives – each one shaped by heartbreaks, breakthroughs and lessons – I'm, hopefully, not even halfway through. While living a long life isn't guaranteed, the average life expectancy for women in the UK is 82.8 years old, so, if I'm lucky, there are still many chapters to come. Some will be totally unknown, and others are inevitable – like perimenopause and menopause. There's still joy to chase, rage to channel, and space to take up. The fight for equality is far from over.

And yet, despite hopefully having so many decades ahead of me, I'm already aware of how the world is beginning to unsee me. I'm already worrying about getting older, even though I know the alternative is death. Even though I know the obsession with female youth is both creepy and outdated and that it comes from a time when a woman's value was measured by her fertility and therefore her age. We might have moved on in theory, but these messages and themes run deep.

Ageing feels like such a gendered double standard. On magazine covers, men are allowed to frown and show their lines as a mark of wisdom and masculinity. By contrast, women's skin is airbrushed so it is unrealistically poreless, smooth and plastic. We are not given the grace of expression or signs of life. Nowhere reflects the double standard of ageing more than Hollywood. By the age of forty, women hold only 20 per cent of leading film roles, compared to 80 per cent for men.[39] In 2019, only 3 per cent of films featured a female lead aged forty-five or older, compared to 25 per cent of major male characters aged forty plus. A *TIME* analysis of 6,000 actors found that men's careers peak around age forty-six,[40] while women's peak at just thirty. Men are allowed to grow into gravitas, playing heroes and romantic leads well into middle age, while women are quietly phased out no matter how adored they were in their twenties and thirties.

Just look at *Top Gun: Maverick*. Tom Cruise returned as Maverick twenty-five years after the original, but Kelly McGillis, who played his love interest, was replaced by a younger actress. Neither McGillis nor Meg Ryan returned, and both were scrutinised in the media and online for how they looked: one mocked for ageing naturally and 'letting herself go', the other criticised for surgery and 'clinging to youth'. How desperate! Meanwhile, George Clooney is celebrated as a *silver fox*. Film and TV don't just reflect double standards, they reinforce them. And if we aren't telling the stories of older women, then they don't just lose visibility but we erase their wisdom, complexity and power. Female youth is so normalised in celebrity relationships that when Keanu Reeves stepped out with his girlfriend Alexandra Grant, the internet gasped at how old she was, despite her being nine years his junior.

Men are given the grace to age into themselves, while women are told not to let ourselves go. Even as we pass out of our fertile years, we're reminded our value still lies in looking good. And if we try to preserve youth? It must look effortless. Be forever twenty-five, but don't try too hard. Don't admit to Botox, but don't actually look old. It's another impossible standard.

I always said I'd grow old gracefully . . . until I started actually growing older. It's confronting. I hate that it is, but it is. In my twenties, I was already afraid of getting older. On my twenty-fifth birthday, I remember feeling like I was on the 'wrong side' of my twenties. I had just left my job to try to make it in television, and the press assumed I was two years younger than I was. I never corrected them, and I felt lucky to have had the years shaven off. I lived in fear of being found out, terrified that if they knew my real age I'd be seen as too old and too irrelevant.

As I approached my thirtieth birthday, I felt a growing sense of dread. I wasn't old enough to be thirty – not when I hadn't ticked off the milestones I thought I was supposed to. No house. No relationship. Definitely no millions in the bank (still deep in my overdraft until I was twenty-nine). I hadn't achieved the things I thought defined success. At school, thirty had felt ancient. I remember making pacts with platonic male friends that, if we hadn't married by then, we'd marry each other – because, apparently, being single at thirty was the worst possible outcome. Better to be in a loveless relationship than to be old and alone!

As the birthday crept closer, I had a full-on breakdown. I felt sad, angry and confused. I worried my career would be over before it had even begun. When my friends threw me a surprise party with giant silver 3-0 balloons, I couldn't enjoy it. Instead of celebrating the people in my life who loved me, I panicked that the media would find out my real age. I felt exposed. Like I'd reached the edge of a cliff, and all that lay ahead was a fast descent into irrelevance, invisibility and decay.

Maybe you're reading this and feel the same dread. If so, I want to tell you this: thirty isn't old. And neither is forty, or fifty, or even sixty. I've found so much reassurance in watching women of all ages live boldly and unapologetically. You'll reach that so-called cliff and find it's not a drop-off – it's a plateau. A place to breathe. The air is clearer. You can appreciate the view. Life slows down, and it gets better.

Now, on the other side of thirty, making my way daily closer to the next big milestone, I'm happier than I've ever been. More confident. More grounded. More *me*. I feel more attractive and sexier than I ever did in my twenties (though, of course, I wish I'd appreciated my younger beauty when I had it). My relationships are deeper, my boundaries stronger. My friends and I are all ageing like fine wine – and we tolerate far less. Maybe that's what makes older women such a threat to the patriarchy: we know who we are, and we're no longer afraid to ask for more.

If our culture didn't distract us with anti-ageing creams and injectables, imagine how powerful we'd be. And what a waste of energy it all is, because we are beautiful at every stage – even if we cannot see it in the moment. As the screenwriter Nora Ephron so eloquently said: 'Anything you think is wrong with your body at the age of thirty-five you will be nostalgic for at the age of forty-five.'

If only we could see lines not as flaws but as markers of wisdom and life – like the Bayeux Tapestry, each one telling stories of joy, sadness, heartbreak and laughter. In nature, we marvel at the lines on a tree trunk. Each ring quietly declares its age and all it has weathered, and yet we never think the tree has lost its beauty. Quite the opposite – we revere it. It stands strong. Grounded. Rooted in time.

But I'm not there. Not yet. Perhaps I'm even complicit. I exfoliate, tone, inject, conceal. I buy the products. I don't promote anything with anti-ageing messaging – I draw that line – but I do use them. My relationship with Botox is particularly complicated. I first invited the poison into my face at thirty. Not because I hated my reflection, but because I was told it was *preventative*. I had two faint lines – one across my forehead and one between my brows. But once the Botox wore off, I swear I had five. Maybe it's because the rest of my face was working overtime in compensation?

I've twice lost my ability to smile after Botox. The irony

hasn't been lost on me that I injected my face to look 'happier' and lost the ability to show happiness in the process. I also love my smile, so in trying to fight one problem, I created another.

I don't love my face full of Botox – it's harsh, frozen, blank. But I don't love it without either. Now I feel trapped. Like Demi Moore's character in her Oscar-winning role in *The Substance* – a woman battling ageing only to find herself consumed by it. The more you fight it, the more it finds you.

It's a paradox. I want to be age-positive, but I also find myself trying to pause the process. I talk about it openly online because I don't want to lie and pretend that serums and sheet masks are responsible for my wrinkle-less skin. I don't want women to think I naturally look this way at my age so that they look at their own ageing skin and wonder what is wrong with them. But sometimes I wonder if honesty is the answer. Does transparency help, or am I just promoting age interventions by normalising them? If the solution to fatphobia is body confidence, then the solution to anti-ageing is ageing. So why do I still struggle to be an age-positive role model?

I follow women online who age boldly and beautifully. Women who go grey, who reject aesthetic pressures, who express themselves without apology. And I genuinely think they are beautiful. So why can't I find that same freedom in myself?

The truth is, in this area, I am not a role model. I'm conflicted. Caught between impossible standards and contradictory messaging. But I *am* certain of one thing: we must stop judging each other for how we choose to age. Because, once again, it's a patriarchal trap and we cannot win. If we fight ageing, we're vain and desperate. If we accept it, we're invisible. Either way, we're punished.

So instead of judging each other, we should be supporting each other however we choose to respond. Because the real enemy is not the woman getting Botox or the one going grey. It's the system that tells us women are no longer valuable or worthy of admiration as the years pass by.

Of course, female ageing isn't just about vanity and looks. I'm thirty-eight, and it wasn't until Davina McCall's documentary that I heard the word 'perimenopause'. That's shocking given that it will affect 50 per cent of the population. I now know it can last up to ten years – an eighth of my life – and I still barely understand it.

Perimenopause is the transitional phase before the point of menopause, marked by fluctuating hormones like oestrogen and progesterone. Symptoms can include irregular periods, fatigue, mood swings, night sweats, anxiety and brain fog. It can begin in your thirties or forties and last years. Menopause itself is defined as the point twelve months after your last period. It lasts just one day – everything after is post-menopause. Treatments like HRT (hormone replacement therapy) can help, yet so many women are either misdiagnosed, dismissed or too embarrassed to ask.

Historically, women going through menopause have often been misunderstood, pathologised or ignored, which speaks volumes about society's discomfort with ageing, female sexuality and women's health – a lethal combination! During the Middle Ages, women were believed to become colder and drier with age due to a humoral imbalance that was thought to cause disease, bitterness or even be the result of witchcraft. During the eighteenth and nineteenth centuries, menopause finally began to be recognised medically, but it was framed as a 'deficiency disease', which caused a loss of femininity, youth and fertility. Many doctors stigmatised it, blaming menopause for hysteria and insanity. For Victorians, menopause was viewed as the beginning of a woman's decline.

While things have drastically improved since then thanks to amazing women like Davina, there is still a long, long way to go. We're still not checking women's hormones, meaning often they have to struggle and push for diagnosis. For two years after having Ada, I felt bone-tired, foggy, drained. I thought I was perimenopausal. But it turned out I had iron-deficiency from childbirth and needed a transfusion. I'd normalised my exhaustion as 'just being a mum'.

Like me, many women still don't know what to expect because of the lack of education around our own bodies. GPs often lack training, with many women still being gaslit or denied hormone replacement therapy (HRT), and perimenopause is still underdiagnosed and undertreated. Like so many other areas of women's health, we need more education, research and investment into menopause. We also need laws to protect older women as they navigate this transition because, despite rising awareness, there is still no specific legal protection for menopausal women in UK workplaces. In 2022, Parliament rejected calls to make menopause a protected characteristic under the Equality Act, and while guidance now encourages employers to support menopausal staff, no policy is legally required. A proposed Employment Rights Bill aims to change this, but at the time of writing it hasn't yet become law.

Until it does, we continue to let down women as they suffer in silence. Once they are no longer seen as sexually or reproductively 'useful' to society, we disempower them and render them invisible. Yet, mature women carry memory, knowledge and truth. We could be the matriarchs of society empowering younger generations of women to expect and demand better. Instead, we're told to disappear. Well, I won't. I intend to grow old loudly. I intend to take up space. To be seen, even when the world stops looking.

A few years ago, I became friends with a woman who was then 97. She stayed my friend until she died at 104. She drank wine every day and told brilliant stories. I asked her what the secret to a long life was, and she said: 'Don't take things so seriously. And fall in love as many times as possible.' She was young at heart until the end. Being around her reminded me that life doesn't end at forty, fifty or eighty. There are still new versions of ourselves to meet. Still people to love.

There are still many chapters left in my story. There's still joy to be felt. Rage to be channelled. Systems to dismantle. But at least, in the next chapter, I won't have to waste any time second-guessing or shrinking myself.

SISTERHOOD
ˈsɪs.tə.hʊd
noun

a strong feeling of friendship and support among women who are involved in action to improve women's rights.

CONCLUSION

Once, I was a two-year-old girl who was loud and who looked at her reflection with awe. I didn't question my worth. I didn't measure my body. I didn't shrink myself to fit inside anyone else's idea of what I should be. But along the journey between girlhood and womanhood, I was slowly taught to be quiet. To be small. To be pleasing. I learned to hate my body. To tie my worth to numbers: the ones on a scale, a waistband, a screen. I was taught that I wasn't a whole, but incomplete until I found another half. I spent so much time trying to make other people like me that I forgot how to like myself. It took me a long time to return to myself. A life coach qualification, a bookshelf full of self-help, a not-so-small fortune in therapy bills.

I still worry about inevitable things, like ageing, like change, and about being the best mum to Alf and Ada. But I no longer seek external validation to feel worthy. I live with purpose. With a strong sense of self-esteem. I might not look in the mirror with the same wonder I did as a child, but I remind myself to zoom out and respect this body for everything it's carried me through.

Now, that little confident girl lives again, this time as my daughter. My greatest hope for her is that she never feels the need to shrink. That she never believes her value lies in her appearance, her weight or her ability to please others. I want her to know the power of her beauty and brains and for her to live a large life, one rooted in confidence, purpose and self-respect. I also want her to know the importance of sisterhood.

To know how to navigate jealousy and to lift other women up, to understand instinctively that the sun never compares itself to the moon. They both shine. Women are not her competition.

I want her to rise above the sexist labels that will try to box her in and keep her small so that she can step into her power, in her career, in her relationships, and, most of all, within herself. I want her to love herself first and most, so that she expects nothing less from anyone else. She will know that rejection and failure are not shameful – because I will tell her they're inevitable and essential. I don't care if she becomes a lawyer or follows her gran's footsteps into hairdressing. I don't care if she chooses motherhood or chooses to be child-free. What matters is that she has the right to choose a life that makes her feel alive. And that she respects the paths of others, even when they look nothing like her own.

As I reflect on my own journey through girlhood and womanhood, I realise how much of my experience is shared. You may not have walked my exact path, but if you've battled with your body, questioned your worth or lived for external approval, then you'll know something about what I mean. Whatever your story, I hope this book reminds you that you are not alone, and that you are enough. I hope it lights a fire in you, not just to heal but to rise. Maybe it helps you reconsider things you'd accepted as natural?

For so long I felt like I had to be a chameleon, trying to change or fix myself to fit into different environments. No matter where I was, or who I was with, I always felt like an outsider. I've used the word 'normal' so much through this book, and in so many situations I've been made to feel that I've failed to hit that standard, that there was something wrong with me, some natural instinct I was lacking. But what I've learned is there is no one way to be normal. Everyone's idea of what is normal is completely unique. And no matter where I've been, whether north or south, upper or working class, at home or boarding school, at a showbusiness event or the school gate, I've seen so many women struggling to fit into the boxes that the world expects them to.

I've learned that the female experience in all of those spaces is uncannily similar. The same messaging holds us back and stops us from being our most confident self no matter where we live or who we are. But do you know what is normal for women?

What's normal is battling against the patriarchy and misogyny. Yes, that might look completely different for women in all different walks of life, but it seems to be inescapable at some point of our life that we will be shamed, stripped of our confidence and minimised simply because we happened to have been born female. I imagine all of you have been called at least one of the derogatory terms woven through the chapters of this book at some point in your lives:

Bossy · Drama Queen · Attention Seeker · Diva · Cow
Prude · Frumpy · Frigid · Dyke · Tart · Slut · Whore · Ho
Pick-Me Girl · Bimbo · Airhead · Posh Totty · Cat Lady · Crazy
Spinster · Feminazi · Bitch · Gold Digger · Needy · Bridezilla
Trophy Wife · WAG · Nag · Ballbuster · Ball and Chain · Mumsy
MILF · Homewrecker · Cougar · Battle Axe · Mutton · Witch
Hysterical · Hag · Matron · Biddy · Bint · Crone

Sometimes to our faces.
Sometimes behind our backs.
Maybe we've used these words to describe other women. I know I have. It has helped my own insecurities to try to bring women down with these words.

People often talk about reclaiming these words by turning them into something empowering, and maybe that works for some. But, personally, I don't want any label that was built to shrink me. I don't believe a sexually liberated woman is a 'slut'. I don't believe a woman who chooses not to have sex is a 'prude'. I believe in something bigger: the right to live without definition. The right to make decisions based on our own likes, wants and desires – rather than shame, ostracisation or fear. I want us to break free of the gendered social constraints that aim to keep us compliant.

These words box us in and make us fear stepping outside of the rigid walls of what is acceptable as a woman. These words are designed to confuse us, divide us, and make us doubt ourselves. We cannot ever beat these words because if we're not one, we're another. And for as long as we remain trapped in these contradictions where we are damned if we do, judged if we don't, we are too busy fighting each other to demand a system that works for us.

A woman who speaks up is a bitch.
A woman who stays quiet is weak.
A woman who enjoys sex is a slut.
A woman who doesn't is frigid.
A woman who dares to discuss politics is a bimbo.
No matter what we do, we're wrong.
And that's the point.
Because if we're busy looking inwards, picking ourselves apart, or looking sidewards, judging other women's choices, if we're too exhausted trying to strike the impossible balance, then we're too busy battling each other to realise the real fight is not with other women but with the conditions that make it so hard to be one.

The antidote? It's not perfection. It's not being the 'right' kind of woman. It's not finding the magical sweet spot between madonna and whore.

It's sisterhood.

Sisterhood means seeing through the trap. Refusing to

judge the woman who breastfeeds *or* the one who uses formula. Refusing to side-eye the woman who's had Botox *or* the one who's letting her grey grow in. Refusing to roll our eyes at the tradwife, the single mum, the child-free woman, the career woman, the stay-at-home mum, the one who wants to marry young, the one who never wants to marry at all.

Sisterhood means understanding that the fight is not between *us*. It's between us and the world that benefits from our division.

That's why feminism must be inclusive. True feminism is about equality not superiority, and certainly not exclusion. It's not about punching down on the rights of others or gatekeeping what it means to be a woman. Trans people are not a threat to womanhood. In fact, they face many of the same oppressions under patriarchy: violence, body policing, shame and systemic neglect. The real threat to all of us is a culture that continues to centre power around cis straight white men. Dividing marginalised groups only serves to uphold that power. If we want to create a more just world, we must stand together.

That's also why intersectional feminism is so essential. White feminism – the kind that centres the experiences of privileged, middle-class white women while ignoring the voices of Black women, working-class women, disabled women and trans women – simply isn't enough. Feminism that doesn't include *all* women is just another form of privilege. If we're truly fighting for equality, then we must fight for everyone.

Whether you want to age naturally or get a Kris Jenner facelift. Stay child-free or be a mum. Be a wife or stay single. We should all have the choice. And a system that supports and protects us no matter what that choice is. Whether we consider ourselves 'feminists' or not, we all benefit from it. In the 1950s everyone was a tradwife. Today we can make the choice to follow traditional gendered norms or not. What feminism has given us is the right to leave an unsafe or unhappy relationship. We all benefit from the generations of women who fought for reproductive rights, gay rights, education, the vote, workplace protection. We owe so much to the women who came before us.

We all want autonomy. We all want freedom. We all want the right to shape our lives in ways that make us feel safe, joyful and full.

So, let's stop calling each other names. Let's stop playing the game that allows so many double standards between men and women. There is no one right way to be a woman.

It's why I try my hardest to support women in all their choices. I don't judge the woman in full glam, and I don't judge the woman who rejects makeup. I don't think a woman should have to justify being child-free any more than one who feels she was born to be a mum. Sleep with who you want. Sleep with no one. Just don't drag another woman down on the way. I'm a girl's girl, a mum's mum, and a woman who believes that feminism means showing up for each other – even when our choices look different.

So be loud. Be bossy. Be unshrinkable. Whether you're sixteen or sixty-six, it's never too late to take up space. To laugh too loudly. To stop apologising. To live a life that is yours – truly and fully.

And, finally, here's what I'll leave you with:
Never speak badly about yourself – or about other women.
Never associate ageing with decline.
Never assume a woman's choices are 'for men'.
Never reward a man for doing the bare minimum.
Never shrink yourself to be digestible.
And always, always remember: if Donald Trump can become president – twice – then you, my friend, can do anything you want to.

ACKNOWLEDGEMENTS

I dedicate this book to women.

The ones who came before us who paved the way, the ones who had to suffer and the ones who were erased from history.

To my mum, who sacrificed so much to make me – in every sense of the word.

And to my sister Joelle, who has always been my best friend.

And to my mother-in-law Clare, you defy all the sexist stereotypes, and I feel so lucky to have you.

To my sister-in-law Kristen for looking over these pages and giving me your words of advice.

To my girlfriends past and present, who picked me up when I had shrunk – Jenny, Wakey, Taylor, Caz, Amelia, Emma, Jas, Steph, Lilah, Charlotte, Jackie, Vicky, Liv and Hannah.

To my guardian angel Josie – I hope you know how eternally grateful I am to you for being my knight in shining armour.

To my mum friends, who helped me to find my pink – Louise, Vix, Robyn, Melissa, Steph and Liv.

And to all the friends I'll make in the next chapter.

To you – who have followed me online and been my friends through all the highs and lows of each chapter of my life.

And to all the women I'll meet in the next chapter.

This is also to the next generation of women, who still have such a fight ahead of them.

Especially my daughter, Ada. I hope you always keep

ACKNOWLEDGEMENTS

your confidence and never let the world convince you to be less than.

To the men who stand up for us – loudly. We appreciate your allyship so much.

To my dad, brother Stuart, father-in-law Mark and, of course, to my partner and coelacanth, Tommy.

And, of course, to my favourite boy in the whole wide world, my son Alfie. I hope one day you read this and know how important it is to always speak up for us.

To all the agents who have ever believed in me and who have helped me get to where I am now. Sal, Chloe, Amy, Mitch, Matt and Steph, and most importantly Dan, the dream-maker, who brought this dream to life.

And to Eve for bringing *Bimbo* to life online and holding the fort.

And, finally, to all the team at Penguin Random House, who made my dream of writing a book come true. Thank you for believing in me and helping me to share *Bimbo* with the world. To Zennor, Alita, Sophie, Jessie, Olivia, Aoifke, Anna, Joanna, Zahraa, Helen, Alice, Emily, Kirsten and Phoenix – thank you. And to Katherine – how would I have done any of this without you? Thank you for the words and encouragement.

How lucky am I to have so many amazing women on Team *Bimbo*?

NOTES

1. Francis Green, 'Private Schools and Inequality', Institute of Fiscal Studies, 2022.
2. Private Education Policy Forum, www.pepf.co.uk.
3. Erez Levon et al, 'Speaking Up: Accents and Social Mobility', The Sutton Trust, 3 November 2022.
4. 'Evidence of Pornography's Influence on Harmful Sexual Behaviour Among Children', Children's Commissioner, 9 May 2023.
5. Mike Males, 'Adult liaison in the "epidemic" of "teenage" birth, pregnancy, and venereal disease', *The Journal of Sex Research*, 1992.
6. Kirstin R. Mitchell et al, 'Why Do Men Report More Opposite-Sex Sexual Partners Than Women? Analysis of the Gender Discrepancy in a British National Probability Survey', National Library of Medicine, 25 July 2018.
7. 'Sexism in Schools Survey', Unison, 2024.
8. 'Sexual Harassment and Sexual Violence in Schools: Government Response to the Committee's Third Report of Session 2016–17', Women and Equalities Select Committee Report, 2016.
9. 'Review of Sexual Abuse in Schools and Colleges', Ofsted, 10 June 2021.
10. NHS Digital, as reported in 'Self-harm hospital admissions up 22% for children aged eight to 17', bbc.co.uk, 23 March 2023.
11. Emla Fitzsimons and Praveetha Patalay, 'Mental ill-health at age 17 in the UK: Prevalence of and inequalities in psychological distress, self-harm and attempted suicide', Centre for Longitudinal Studies, 2020.

12 UK Parliament, 'Rape: Prosecutions', Hansard, Volume 843, debated on Thursday, 30 January 2025.
13 Ministry of Justice, 'The end-to-end rape review report on findings and actions', 18 June 2021.
14 'Sex attack victims usually know attacker, says new study', BBC, 1 March 2018.
15 Office for National Statistics, 2021.
16 Allen Gabriel et al, 'Cellulite: Current Understanding and Treatment', National Library of Medicine, 2023.
17 Office for National Statistics, 2024.
18 Paul Dolan, *Happy Ever After: Escaping The Myth of The Perfect Life* (Allen Lane, 2019).
19 'Rise of the SHEconomy', Morgan Stanley, 23 September 2019.
20 Catherine Gray, *The Unexpected Joy of Being Single: Locating unattached happiness* (Aster, 2018).
21 Office for National Statistics, 2016.
22 Victor Pino et al, 'The effects of aging on semen parameters and sperm DNA fragmentation', National Library of Medicine, 2020.
23 M. S. Oud et al, 'A de novo paradigm for male infertility', Nature Communications, 2022.
24 Hagai Levine et al, 'Temporal trends in sperm count: a systematic review and meta-regression analysis', National Library of Medicine, 2017.
25 Thomas G. Travison et al, 'Temporal trends in testosterone levels and treatment in older men', National Library of Medicine, 2009.
26 Paolo Capogrosso et al, 'Age at First Presentation for Erectile Dysfunction: Analysis of Changes over a 12-yr Period', National Library of Medicine, 2019.
27 Niels E. Skakkebaek et al, 'Male Reproductive Disorders and Fertility Trends: Influences of Environment and Genetic Susceptibility', National Library of Medicine, 2015.
28 Richard Fry et al, 'In a Growing Share of U.S. Marriages, Husbands and Wives Earn About the Same', Pew Research, 13 April 2023.
29 UK Health Security Agency, 2018.

NOTES

30 Unicef UK.
31 Diane Wiessinger et al, *Sweet Sleep – Nighttime and Naptime Strategies for the Breastfeeding Family,* La Lêche League International, 28 November 2018.
32 'Saving Lives, Improving Mothers' Care 2024 – Lessons learned to inform maternity care from the UK and Ireland Confidential Enquiries into Maternal Deaths and Morbidity 2020–22', MBRRACE – UK, October 2024.
33 Office for National Statistics, 2023.
34 Siobhan Quenby et al, 'Miscarriage matters: the epidemiological, physical, psychological, and economic costs of early pregnancy loss', *The Lancet,* 1 May 2021.
35 ChannelMum.com/The Baby Show, 2019.
36 YouGov, 2021.
37 Royal College of Midwives.
38 Femicide Census, 2020.
39 'Why the Age of 40 is so important in Hollywood', *Washington Post,* 19 September 2016.
40 'Hollywood's Glaring Gender Gap', *TIME,* October 2015.

READING LIST

Attached: Are you Anxious, Avoidant or Secure? How the science of adult attachment can help you find – and keep – love, Amir Levine and Rachel S. F. Heller (Bluebird, 2019)

Block, Delete, Move On: It's Not You, It's Them, LalalaLetMeExplain (Bantam Press, 2022)

Boarding School Syndrome: The Psychological Trauma of the 'Privileged Child', Joy Schaverien (Routledge, 2015)

Essays in Love, Alain de Boton (Picador, 2006)

Fix the System, Not the Woman, Laura Bates (Simon & Schuster, 2022)

Hags: The Demonisation of Middle-Aged Women, Victoria Smith (Fleet, 2023)

Hold on to Your Kids: Why Parents Matter, Gordon Neufeld and Gabor Maté (Knopf, 2024)

Housewife, Ann Oakley (Allen Lane, 1974)

I Feel Bad About My Neck: And Other Thoughts On Being a Woman, Nora Ephron (Vintage, 2006)

In Defence of Witches: Why women are still on trial, Mona Chollet (Picador, 2022)

Matrescence: On the Metamorphosis of Pregnancy, Childbirth and Motherhood, Lucy Jones (Allen Lane, 2023)

The 5 Love Languages: The Secret to Love That Lasts, Gary Chapman (1992)

The Feminine Mystique, Betty Friedan (W. W. Norton, 1963)

READING LIST

The Science of Parenting: How Today's Brain Research Can Help You Raise Happy, Emotionally Balanced Children, Margot Sunderland (Dorling Kindersley, 2006)

The Second Sex, Simone de Beauvoir (1949)

The Unexpected Joy of Being Single: Locating unattached happiness, Catherine Gray (Aster, 2018)

The Woman They Could Not Silence: One woman, her incredible fight for freedom, and the men who tried to make her disappear, Kate Moore (Scribe, 2021)

Wedded Wife: A Feminist History of Marriage, Rachel Lennon (Aurum, 2023)

INDEX

Abercrombie & Fitch, 105–7
Ada (daughter), 1, 18–21, 25, 53, 226–7, 255–7, 293–5, 330–31
ageing, 321–8
Alfie (son), 18, 20–21, 138, 224–8, 230, 243–5, 257, 265–6, 279, 286, 293–5, 301, 305–6, 313, 317
American Pie (film), 63, 67
Andrews, Tommy, 190–93, 202, 203–8, 213, 227, 230, 255–6, 270–72, 301
  parenting and, 277–87, 292
Attached (Levine & Heller), 182
attachment theory, 182–3
Austen, Jane, 204

Baker Brown, Dr Isaac, 251
ball and chain: definition, 194
'banter', 73, 75, 89, 91–2
Barks, Samantha, 119
BBC Radio Cumbria, 106
beauty standards, 52–6

BEBO (social media site), 113
bimbo, 9–12
  definition, 9
Birtley witches, 155–6
body hair, 64, 75
Body Mass Index (BMI), 137
bossy, 14, 24–6, 50
  definition, 14
Botox, 324–5
breasts, 123–9
Bridget Jones (film series), 131
Brontë Sisters, 47

calories, 136
capitalism, 5–6
Cat Lady, 155–8
  definition, 154
Celebrity Big Brother (TV programme), 177–81
cellulite, 134–5
Chapman, Dr Gary, 183–4
Charles III, King of the United Kingdom, 200

INDEX

childbirth, 236–7, 241–7, 248, 251–2, 253–7, 258–68
  'baby weight', 259–60
  caesarean sections, 253–7
  faecal incontinence, 265–6
  maternity care, 248–9, 254–5
  pain-relief and, 247, 248, 251
  pelvic prolapse, 263–4
  postnatal depression, 292–3, 295–6, 301–3
  postpartum recovery, 236–40, 258–68, 270–76
  pregnancy, 211–12, 221–2, 236–40
  sex after childbirth, 270–76
  urinary incontinence, 265
  see also motherhood; parenting
childcare, 230, 233–4, 288–90, 305–6
children, 18–23
  assertion and, 24–6
  boys, 313–17
  gendered dressing, 20–22
  menstruation and, 40–43
  sexualised games, 37–9, 59
  toys, 22
  see also schools
clitoridectomy, 251
Clooney, George, 322
clothing, 127–8, 136
Couzens, Wayne, 92

Covid-19 pandemic 208, 213–14, 244, 294–5
crazy, 102, 104, 251
  definition, 100
Cruise, Tom, 322

de Beauvoir, Simone, 48
diet culture, 130–39
divorce, 160–61
drama queen: definition, 77
dyke: definition, 111

Edwards, Rick, 120
Elizabeth II, Queen of the United Kingdom, 199
Ellis-Bextor, Sophie, 228
engagement rings, 200
Ephron, Nora, 324
Esquire magazine, 145
Everard, Sarah, 91–2
Everyone's Invited (charity), 74

fatherhood *see* parenting
fatphobia, 130–39
female anatomy, education and, 75–6
Feminine Mystique, The (Friedan), 298
femininity, 3, 10, 49–51, 88–90, 120–22
feminism, 2, 6–7, 163, 168–9, 286, 334–5

INDEX

fertility, 165–7, 236
film industry, 321–2
Five Love Languages, The (Chapman), 183–4
Flack, Caroline, 302
Foden, Phil, 91
football supporters, 91
France, 33, 266
French Connection, 118–19
Freud, Sigmund, 61–2
Friedan, Betty, 298
Friends (TV series), 131
friendship groups, 171, 174–6
frigid: definition, 58

gender equality, 6–7
   clothing, 127–8
   see also gender stereotyping
gender norms, 18–23, 26
gender pay gap, 160
gender stereotyping, 50, 89
gender-based violence, 314–15
Gibson, Josie, 144–5
'girlfriend material', 61, 89
GQ magazine, 145
Grant, Alexandra, 322
Gray, Catherine, 165

hag: definition, 320
Hale, Sir Matthew, 197
Harry, Prince, Duke of Sussex, 200

Heller, Rachel S. F., 182
Hillingdon, Lady Alice, 276
homophobia, 22–3
homosexuality, 113–16
HRT (hormone replacement therapy), 326–7
hypnobirthing, 242
hysterectomy, 251
hysterical, 249–51
   definition, 235

'incel' culture, 315
internalised misogyny, 50–51, 63
Ireland, 160
Itsu, 107

James, Ashley
   accent, 31–3
   ageing and, 322–8
   anxious attachment and, 182–3
   birth and childhood, 15–17, 184–5
   boarding school (prep), 27–35, 37–41
   boarding school (secondary), 47–51, 59–60, 65–7, 71–3, 123–4
   body dysmorphia, 121–2
   boobs, 123–9, 133
   breakdown, 79–80
   celebrity and, 120–22, 125
   cheating and, 93–4, 101–4

James, Ashley – *cont'd*
  childbirth, 241–9, 253–7, 261–4, 270–76
  children and, 212–13
  clothing, 127–8, 133, 136
  dating scene and, 152, 188–91
  diving course, 170–71
  DJing, 171, 295
  exercise and, 132, 137
  father, 16, 29–30, 33–5, 54, 178, 181, 197–8, 215
  feminism and, 168–9, 178, 219–20
  first jobs, 97–9
  friends, 171, 174–5, 188
  London and, 304–5
  loneliness, 174–6, 188
  loses virginity, 66–7
  love and affection and, 185–7
  low self-esteem, 104, 145, 147
  marriage and, 159, 195–202, 205–8
  mental health, 301–2, 304, 323
  Mexico, 152–3, 169–70
  modelling, 52, 105–6, 124–6, 133–5, 168
  money and, 178–9
  mother, 16, 29–30, 33–5, 54, 131, 151, 178, 181, 184–5, 215
  motherhood and, 7, 138, 166, 175, 211–40, 256, 274–5, 277–9, 292–300, 306–12
  pregnancy, 238–40, 242
  primary school, 24
  relationships, 78–9, 90–94, 101–3, 112–13, 143–9, 184, 193, 270, 277–87
  self-confidence, 2, 5, 7–8, 24–6, 59, 106, 144–7
  self-harm and, 80–81
  sense of injustice, 118
  sexual assault, 82–7
  sexuality and, 113–16
  single status, 170–72, 175
  social media and, 126–7, 134–5, 168
  sports and, 124
  television industry and, 107–10, 117–18
  university, 88, 92–3, 97, 106
  weight and, 130–39, 259
Jane Eyre (Charlotte Brontë), 47
Jeremy Vine Show, The (TV programme), 226
Johnson, Boris, 200, 208

language, 3–4, 6, 8
  derogatory terms for women, 332–4
learned behaviours, 18
'left on the shelf', 150–53
Levine, Amir, 182
Lewis, Martin, 205
LGBTQ+ community, 115
life expectancy, 321

INDEX

Locke, Ollie, 110, 112–13
'locker-room talk', 91–2
London, 304–5
loneliness, 174–6
love, 78–9, 185–7

Made in Chelsea (TV reality show), 107–10, 117, 120
'madonna-whore complex', 4, 58, 61–3
male superiority, 49
'manosphere', 315
marriage, 143, 150–51, 159–64, 195–202, 204–7, 250
   arranged marriages, 204
   coverture, 197
   men and, 163, 200–202
   weddings, 198–201
maternal mental load, 280–82
matrescence, 306–8
McCall, Davina, 326–7
McGillis, Kelly, 322
'mean girls', 51, 54–5
menopause, 326–7
menstruation, 40–43, 250
Merabi, Nadine, 128
MILF: definition, 269
Mills, Scott, 106
misogyny, 91–2, 315–16
modelling, 105–6
Moore, Demi, 325
Morgan Stanley, 163

Moss, Kate, 131
motherhood, 7–8, 18–19, 175, 211–34, 236–40, 280, 309–12
   boys and, 313–17
   breastfeeding, 224–8, 232–3
   childcare, 230, 233–4, 288–90, 305–6
   fertility and, 165–7
   judgement and, 231–4
   marriage and, 162–3
   maternal mental health, 301–3
   matrescence, 306–8
   motherhood regret, 297–300
   'mum guilt', 288–90
   sleep and, 228–30
   see also childbirth; parenting
Moyles, Chris, 106
'mum guilt', 288–90
mumsy, 219
   definition, 210

nag: definition, 291
needy: definition, 173
nepotism, 5
Netherlands, 267
Newcastle, 156

objectification of women, 53, 123–9
Ockenden Report, 248, 254
Ockenden, Donna, 248

INDEX

Only Way Is Essex, The (TV series), 132

Paltrow, Gwyneth, 131
parenting, 22, 176, 277–87, 288–90, 299, 311–12
   household chore division, 282–7
   maternal mental load, 280–82
   see also motherhood
patriarchy, 5–6, 195–9
Pelicot, Gisèle, 87
Pelvic Girdle Pain (PGP), 238–9
perimenopause, 326–7
Philip, Prince, Duke of Edinburgh, 199, 200
Pick-Me Girl, 89–90
   definition, 46
politics, 10–12
pornography, 69–70, 76
'pretty privilege', 52–6
Pride and Prejudice (Austen), 204
'princesses', 19–20
promiscuity, 61–3

racism, 5–6
rape, 85–7
Raphael, Dana, 306
reality television, 107–8, 177
'red flags', 186–7
Reeves, Keanu, 322
regional accents, 31–3

relationships, 149, 159
   childbirth and, 278–9
   love and, 204
   parenting and, 277–87
religion, 5, 62, 199, 253
Ryan, Meg, 322

Salem, Massachusetts, 155
same-sex relationships, 113–16
Sara, Soma, 74
schools
   boarding school syndrome, 28
   private education, 27–35
   sexism and sexual violence in, 71–4
   sexist bullying, 75–6
Second Sex (de Beauvoir), 48
self-harm, 80
sex, 67–8, 69–70, 236–8, 276
   after childbirth, 270–76
   consent and, 70
   female orgasm, 90–91
   sex drive, 63
   sex education, 67
   shame and, 70
   teenage sex, 67–8
   'tight vaginas', 236–7
sexism, 73–4, 91–2
sexual assault, 82–7
sexual independence, 62–3
sexualisation, 59–60, 64, 120–27
sexualised insults, 37, 57–61

INDEX

sexuality, 113–15
Shallow Hal (film), 131
Simpson, Jessica, 131
single men, 176
single women, 155–8, 159, 162–4
sisterhood, 333–4
  definition, 329
slavery, 250
slut, 59–61
  definition, 57
  slut-shaming, 60–64, 73, 127, 226
social class, 5–6, 29–34, 72
social conditioning, 15–17
social inequality, 27–8
social media, 289–90, 315
Spencer, Charles, 28
spinster, 157–8
  definition, 142
  see also single women
Steph's Packed Lunch (TV programme), 227
Substance, The (film), 325
suicide, 301–3
Swift, Taylor, 63, 162

tart: definition, 36
teenagers
  teenage pregnancies, 62
  teenage relationships, 67–8
This Morning (TV programme), 11, 128, 205

Top Gun: Maverick (film), 322
toxic masculinity, 314–17
Trump, Donald, 91, 200, 335

UK government policy, 11, 12, 252, 315, 327
Unexpected Joy of Being Single, The (Gray), 165
University Radio Nottingham, 106

vaginal mesh scandal, 249
vaginismus, 273
Vance, J. D., 155
victim blaming, 19, 85–7
Victoria, Queen of the United Kingdom, 200

Waddingham, Hannah, 128
'weaponised incompetence', 281
Weber, Bruce, 105
Whiley, Jo, 106
white supremacy, 5–6, 52
whore: definition, 96
William, Prince of Wales, 200
Willis, Emma, 179
witches, 155–6
'woke', 6
women's health, 248–52
women's rights, 160–62
women's suffrage, 157

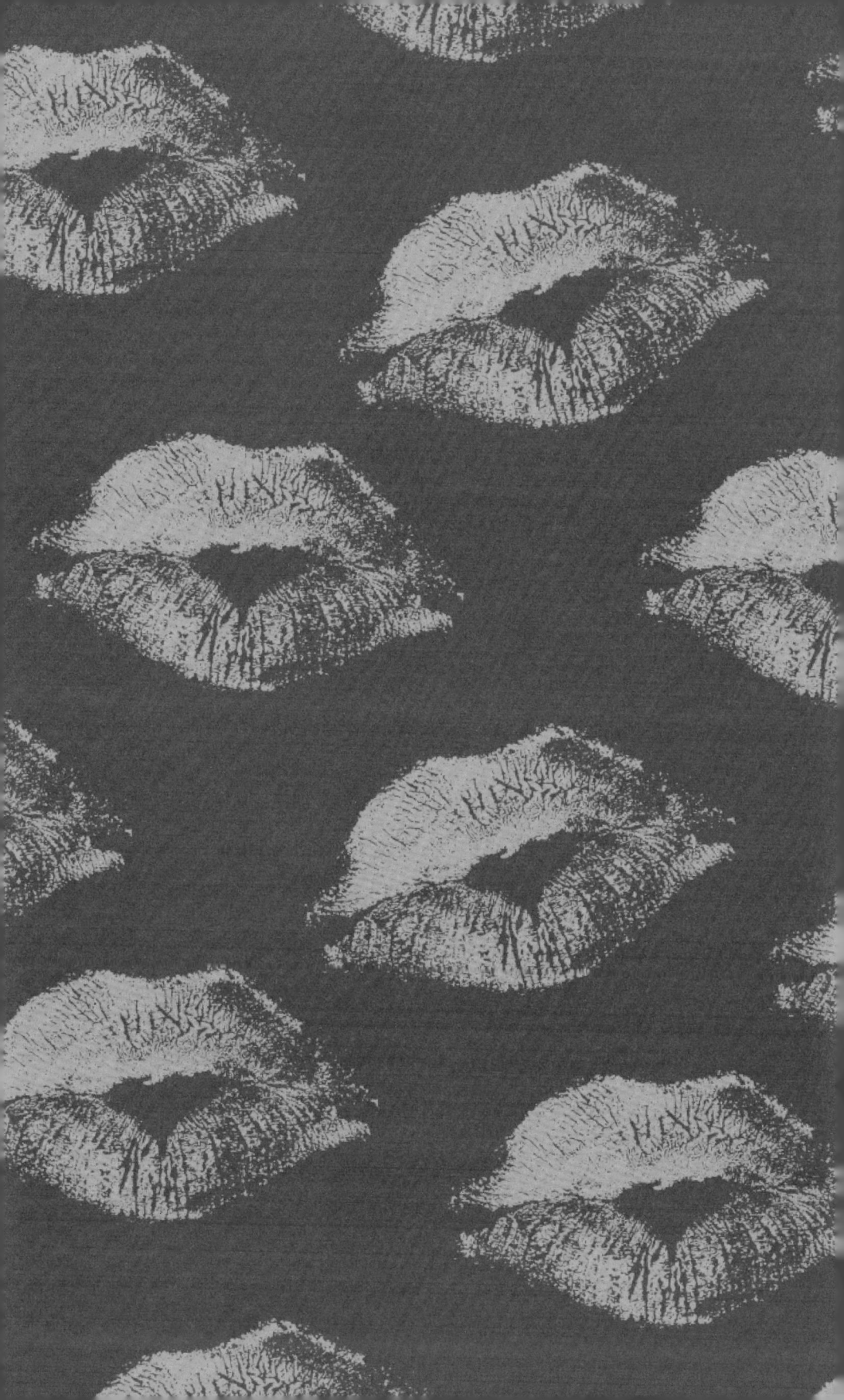